Handbook of Acoustic Accessibility

Best Practices for Listening, Learning, and Literacy in the Classroom

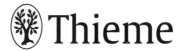

Handbook of Acoustic Accessibility
Best Practices for Listening, Learning, and Literacy in the Classroom

Joseph J. Smaldino, PhD
Professor Emeritus
University of Northern Iowa
Professor of Audiology
Department of Communication Sciences and Disorders
Illinois State University
Normal, Illinois

Carol Flexer, PhD, CCC-A, LSLS Cert. AVT
Distinguished Professor Emeritus, Audiology
The University of Akron
Akron, Ohio

Thieme
New York · Stuttgart

Thieme Medical Publishers, Inc.
333 Seventh Ave.
New York, NY 10001

Acquisitions Editor: Emily Ekle
Editorial Director,
  Clinical Reference: Michael Wachinger
Senior Vice President, International
  Marketing and Sales: Cornelia Schulze
President: Brian D. Scanlan
Compositor: Prairie Papers Inc.
Editorial Assistant: Chris Malone

Production Editor: Kenneth L. Chumbley
International Production Director:
  Andreas Schabert
Vice President, Finance and Accounts:
  Sarah Vanderbilt
Cover Illustration: Courtesy of Phonak
Printer: Sheridan Books, Inc.

Library of Congress Cataloging-in-Publication Data
Handbook of acoustic accessibility : best practices for listening, learning, and literacy in the classroom / [edited by] Joseph Smaldino, Carol Flexer.
     p. ; cm.
  Includes bibliographical references.
  ISBN 978-1-60406-765-1 (alk. paper)
  I. Smaldino, Joseph J. II. Flexer, Carol Ann.
  [DNLM: 1. Acoustics—instrumentation. 2. Audiology—instrumentation. 3. Educational Technology—instrumentation. 4. Hearing Aids. 5. Hearing. 6. Learning. WV 270]
  617.8—dc23
                                                                                    2011053259

Important note: Medical knowledge is ever-changing. As new research and clinical experience broaden our knowledge, changes in treatment and drug therapy may be required. The authors and editors of the material herein have consulted sources believed to be reliable in their efforts to provide information that is complete and in accord with the standards accepted at the time of publication. However, in view of the possibility of human error by the authors, editors, or publisher of the work herein or changes in medical knowledge, neither the authors, editors, nor publisher, nor any other party who has been involved in the preparation of this work, warrants that the information contained herein is in every respect accurate or complete, and they are not responsible for any errors or omissions or for the results obtained from use of such information. Readers are encouraged to confirm the information contained herein with other sources. For example, readers are advised to check the product information sheet included in the package of each drug they plan to administer to be certain that the information contained in this publication is accurate and that changes have not been made in the recommended dose or in the contraindications for administration. This recommendation is of particular importance in connection with new or infrequently used drugs.

Some of the product names, patents, and registered designs referred to in this book are in fact registered trademarks or proprietary names even though specific reference to this fact is not always made in the text. Therefore, the appearance of a name without designation as proprietary is not to be construed as a representation by the publisher that it is in the public domain.

Printed in the United States of America

5 4 3 2 1

ISBN 978-1-60406-765-1
eISBN 978-1-60406-766-8

While this handbook includes some of the finest writers and thinkers in the area of classroom acoustic accessibility, two are prominently missing: Carl Crandell and Gail Gegg Rosenberg. Even though they are no longer with us, their enthusiasm and advocacy for improving classroom acoustic conditions is a continuing inspiration to us all. Carl and Gail, this one's for you.

Joseph J. Smaldino
DeKalb, Illinois

Carol Flexer
Kent, Ohio

Contents

Preface

Denes and Pinson (1993) in their book, *The Speech Chain: The Physics and Biology of Spoken Language*, describe the elements involved in the sending and receiving of spoken language. These authors eloquently describe the damage to speech perception that can result from a faulty transmission of the speech signal from sender to receiver. In brief, the entire speech chain is disrupted. In a classroom, where accurate speech reception and perception are essential precursors to listening, literacy, and learning, faulty transmission of the speech signal cannot be tolerated and if it is, it might very well be thought of as depriving the student access to the very signal important for education–speech. It is in this context that we decided to focus this handbook on the acoustic conditions, therapies, and technologies that assist in making the speech signal audible, undistorted, and accessible to every student in a classroom. In this regard, acoustic accessibility is akin to "universal design." This term, coined by the architect Ronald L. Mace (1991), refers to ideas meant to produce buildings and environments that are inherently accessible to both people without disabilities and people with disabilities. Universal design ideas applied to classrooms result in acoustic accessibility to speech, and that is how we arrived at a title for the handbook.The topical content was chosen to reflect current practices and technologies designed to maximize the availability of the classroom speech signal for every child.

In the first chapter, the father of acoustic access, Mark Ross, offers an historical perspective as he details his personal encounters with the concept of auditory access as they emerged over the past fifty-five years.

Chapter 2 provides an understanding of the neurological underpinnings of the development of the auditory linguistic system and how such relates to effective and efficient listening in the classroom environment. Chapter 3, which deals with speech perception in the classroom, builds upon the neurological underpinnings and develops a clear and complete basis for why room acoustics, specifically background noise and reverberation, are so harmful to accurate speech perception. Chapter 4, which deals with room acoustics, ANSI standards, and handheld measurement devices, focuses on the most current classroom acoustic standards and provides a methodology for determining compliance with the standard using traditional approaches and inexpensive smart phone technology. Chapter 5 reviews Classroom Audio Distribution System (CADS) literature and brings the reader up-to-date-on the research primarily designed to investigate the efficacy of this popular and widespread technology for improving classroom acoustic conditions. Chapter 6, on current CADS systems, discusses available technologies and presents advantages, disadvantages, and practical considerations for each. Chapter 7, which discusses best practices involving the American Academy of Audiology (AAA) Clinical Practice Guidelines for Hearing Assistance Technology (HAT), overviews the recently completed position statement of the AAA concerning the many varieties of amplification devices utilized in the classroom. Chapter 8, on approaches to functional verification of classroom accessibility, provides a behavioral approach to documenting the effectiveness of classroom modifications (physical or technological). Finally, Chapter 9, on acoustic accessibility and the role of the clinical audiologist, describes how audiologists outside the school structure contribute to acoustic accessibility both within and outside the classroom environment.

All of the authors have designed their chapters to function as a handbook. In this way, we hoped to develop a concise and comprehensible reference that can be readily available for the busy professional, parent, teacher, or other interested individual. The smaller format also allowed us to publish the information faster and to keep the handbook modestly priced. We have attempted, therefore, to create a comprehensive, current and affordable reference for those who strive to make listening and learning a priority for all children, with or without hearing loss, in or outside of the school setting. As always, this handbook reflects a "labor of love" for all those involved. It is our sincere hope that the thoughts and ideas in these pages will assist the reader in their labor of love—the children under their care.

References

Denes, P., & Pinson, E. (1993). *The speech chain: the physics and biology of spoken language.* New York: W.H. Freeman and Company.

Mace, R., Hardie, G., & Place, J. (1991). Accessible environments: toward universal design. In Vischer, J., & Whilte, E. (Eds.), *Design interventions: toward a more humane architecture.* New York: Van Nostrand Reinhold.

Authors

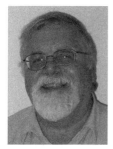

Dr. Joseph J. Smaldino received his doctoral degree from the University of Florida. He is a professor emeritus at the University of Northern Iowa and is currently a professor of audiology in the Department of Communication Sciences and Disorders at Illinois State University. His research areas are hearing aids, speech perception, and audiologic rehabilitation, but he has focused for the last 20 years on the effects of classroom acoustics on listening and learning. He served on the American National Standards Working groups that developed and subsequently revised a national classroom acoustic standard in 2002, 2009, and 2010. He has published extensively in the area and is a long-standing advocate for desirable classroom acoustics and acoustic accessibility. He is the current Editor of *The Volta Review*, one of the oldest research journals in the area of hearing. He has won a distinguished scholar award, has been a Fulbright Research Scholar in Poland, and, in 2011, received the Mauldin Award for individuals who have demonstrated unsurpassed dedication to excellence in education and professionalism in the hearing health care industry, and who have unselfishly giving back to the profession, the community, and the hearing impaired.

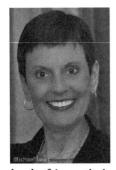

Carol Flexer received her doctorate in audiology from Kent State University in 1982. She was at the University of Akron for 25 years as a distinguished professor of audiology in the School of Speech-Language Pathology and Audiology. Her special areas of expertise include pediatric and educational audiology. Dr. Flexer continues to lecture extensively nationally and internationally about pediatric audiology issues and has authored more than 155 publications. She has coedited and authored twelve books: *Handbook of Acoustic Accessibility; Children with Hearing Loss: Developing Listening and Talking, Birth to Six*, 1st and 2nd eds.; *Pediatric Audiology: Diagnosis, Technology, and Management; Pediatric Audiology Casebook; The Sound of Learning—Why Self-Amplification Matters; How the Student with Hearing Loss Can Succeed in College*, 1st and 2nd eds.; *Sound-Field Amplification: Theory and Practical Applications*, 1st and 2nd eds.; and *Facilitating Hearing and Listening in Young Children*, 1st and 2nd eds. Dr. Flexer is a past president of the Educational Audiology Association, a past president of the American Academy of Audiology, and a past president of the Alexander Graham Bell Association for the Deaf and Hard of Hearing Academy for Listening and Spoken Language. Dr. Flexer is a certified auditory-verbal therapist (LSLS Cert. AVT) and a licensed audiologist. For her research and advocacy for children with hearing loss, Dr. Flexer has received three prestigious awards: two from The Alexander Graham Bell Association for the Deaf and Hard of Hearing—the Volta Award and Professional of the Year Award; and one from the American Academy of Audiology—the 2012 Distinguished Achievement Award. Dr. Flexer also is a certified laughter leader.

Contributors

Karen L. Anderson, PhD
Director
Supporting Success for Children
   with Hearing Loss
Minneapolis, Minnesota

Douglas L. Beck, AuD
Director of Professional Relations
Oticon Inc.
Somerset, New Jersey
Web Content Editor
American Academy of Audiology
Reston, Virginia

Arthur Boothroyd, PhD
Distinguished Professor
   Emeritus
Department of Speech and
   Hearing Sciences
Graduate Center, City
   University of New York
New York, New York

**Carol Flexer, PhD, CCC-A,
   LSLS Cert. AVT**
Distinguished Professor
   Emeritus, Audiology
The University of Akron
Akron, Ohio

Andrew B. John, PhD
Assistant Professor
Department of Communication
   Sciences and Disorders
University of Oklahoma Health
   Sciences Center
Oklahoma City, Oklahoma

Cheryl DeConde Johnson, EdD
The ADEvantage
Leadville, Colorado

Brian M. Kreisman, PhD
Associate Professor
Department of Audiology,
   Speech-Language Pathology,
   and Deaf Studies
Towson University
Towson, Maryland

**Jane R. Madell, PhD, CCC-A/SLP,
   LSLS Cert AVT**
Director
Pediatric Audiology Consulting
New York, New York

Daniel Ostergren, AuD
Consulting Audiologist
Audiology Resources, LLC
Fort Collins, Colorado

Mark Ross, PhD
Professor Emeritus
Communication Sciences
University of Connecticut
Storrs, Connecticut

Joseph J. Smaldino, PhD
Professor Emeritus
University of Northern Iowa
Professor of Audiology
Department of Communication
    Sciences and Disorders
Illinois State University
Normal, Illinois

1 Acoustic Access: An Historical Perspective

Mark Ross

In auditory access considerations, it is necessary to include every link in the communication chain, from the signal source to the nature of the sound signal being delivered to the ear canal (or electrodes for cochlear implants). Any degradation in the signal arising from any link in this chain will affect acoustic access for a listener who is hearing impaired. Thus, poor microphone technique influences acoustic access just as noisy and reverberant rooms or poorly selected hearing aids do. This orientation is in keeping with our overriding goal, which is to deliver the best auditory signal possible consistent with the nature of a person's hearing loss. While we are very sensitive to this goal now, and are much more aware of factors that may interfere with it, it was not always this way. There has been a growing awareness over the years, in part fostered by technological developments. In the following pages, I would like to review some of my personal encounters with the concept of auditory access over the past 55 years.

◆ Early Classrooms

In 1964–1965, an outbreak of maternal rubella significantly increased the incidence of hearing loss in our society. Clinical and educational settings were ill prepared to deal with these newly identified child victims. At the time, virtually no pre-school programs existed for such children except for those in residential schools for the deaf; however, parents wanted their children in day programs close to their homes. Thus, there was a pressing need to find appropriate locations to house such programs within the various communities. Our society responded by making unused classrooms in older schools, church basements, community centers, and other locations available to house pre-school classes. The parents and teachers accepted what was graciously offered and gave little thought to the acoustical conditions existing in the various settings. I consulted in several these programs and visited many more. An early experience I had in one of these classrooms highlights the issue of acoustic accessibility faced by the children who were being educated in these programs.

I was standing a few feet in front of the teacher trying to engage her in conversation. In the meantime, the children were happily and noisily playing in the background. I could barely understand her; the noise level generated by the children was simply too great. As she talked, I kept asking her to repeat. Now, if I, with excellent language abilities, could barely *comprehend* her speech, how in the world would it be possible for those children to *develop* their audition-based linguistic skills when exposed to the same degraded verbal signal? Well, the obvious answer is that they could not and probably did not. They were likely forced into a visual communication mode (speech reading in that setting) or, more likely, never realized their linguistic potential. We know that young children possess an innate capacity to develop language, *provided* the signals they receive are as clear, consistent, and distinctive as possible and are associated with ongoing meaningful experiences. This was not happening in that class. Furthermore, my experience in this setting was not a fluke; I found more or less the same difficulty in just about every pre-school program I visited. In that particular room, located in a church basement, the walls, floor, and ceiling were bare concrete, softened by acoustically meaningless colorful posters and decorations. The offending surfaces were different in the programs located in old schools; those generally included charming wood panels on the walls (at least in New England), large windows, and hard ceilings. Still, while these places may have been visually attractive, acoustically they were something of a nightmare.

Here was another reminder of how acoustic conditions can affect speech and language recognition and development for someone with a hearing loss. Not that I needed a reminder: most of the people I saw as a clinical audiologist complained about understanding speech in noise. Of course, as someone with a long-standing hearing loss, I experienced it myself for many years. My experiences with the children motivated me to further investigate the topic of room acoustics and their effects upon speech perception. It quickly became apparent that poor acoustical conditions were not limited to pre-schools. Little or no acoustical treatment could be found in most typical classrooms; average noise levels often exceeded 50 or 60 dBA and the usual reverberation times were in excess of one second. There were many internal and external noise sources, from bubbling fish tanks, noisy heating and air conditioning systems, chair and table legs scraping the wooden floors, to loud hallway or traffic noises entering the classroom. Often it was difficult for the hearing children to even understand the teacher, a problem that was exacerbated for children with a hearing loss or attention deficit disorder. At the time, noisy and reverberant classrooms seemed an educational non-issue and were essentially ignored, particularly as most of the normally hearing children appeared to comprehend the teacher most of the time. If a child did not respond appropriately or acted up, the behavior was simply dismissed as personal deviant behavior and treated that way. For many years, therefore, children were (and still are, in too many places) deprived of the full benefits of the auditory sense, with consequent repercussions on every aspect of their lives.

◆ Early Chapters and Articles about Acoustic Access

When Dr. Jack Katz invited me to write several chapters in the first edition of *The Handbook of Clinical Audiology*, I used the opportunity to further investigate the impact of acoustical conditions in classrooms by selecting classroom acoustics and speech perception (Ross, 1972) as one of the topics I wrote about. As I went through our professional literature, it was apparent that there were no articles dealing with the behavior of sound in a room and its impact on children. Thus, there were no articles dealing with such basic concepts, from today's perspective, as reverberation time and critical distance. To find any technical material, I had to consult the literature from architectural acoustics. What could be found in the educational and clinical literature were several studies (mostly from Europe) that looked at speech perception as a function of distance from the source and whether a room was untreated or acoustically treated. Thus, these were the studies reviewed and discussed in that initial chapter.

The general results of these studies can be easily summarized: speech perception scores almost always improved the closer the subjects were to the sound source, and regardless of distance, scores were higher in sound-treated as opposed to untreated rooms. As we know now, decreasing the distance from the source boosts the signal to noise (S/N) ratio, still perhaps the most important factor underlying speech perception. Sound-treated rooms, on the other hand, by reducing reflected noise levels, also produce an improved S/N ratio. With either step, increasing the signal level or decreasing the noise, the children's auditory access is improved. The better the children can hear a teacher, the more likely it is that their educational performance will improve. Although they are obvious now, little attention was paid at the time to the full implications of these results. Now, however, classroom acoustics and its effects upon children is a subject area found in many communication disorders training curricula. So we have come a long way, though we undoubtedly still have a ways to go.

Sometimes, however, it is just not practical for a teacher to remain close to a child, or for a classroom to be acoustically treated. Some other way had to be found to improve the S/N ratio of the signal being delivered to a child. Then in the late 1960s and early 1970s personal FM systems were introduced for classroom use. It was apparent that their usage could improve the S/N ratio: by means of a close-talking microphone, the child's "ear" is effectively being moved closer to the teacher. Up to this time (and for a long time afterward), the sound systems used in classrooms were either hard-wired or induction loop systems. The way they were generally used created practical problems in achieving the goal of a favorable S/N ratio.

Almost always there was one microphone, ordinarily located in front of the room a few feet from the teacher, or perhaps suspended from the ceiling. If the teacher moved close to the microphone, the system was perfectly capable of delivering an appropriately high S/N ratio to the children. The problem, however, was that usually the microphone stayed in place while the teacher roamed around the classroom. Unfortunately, even when the teacher was close to the mike, its location at a distance from the children prevented them from effectively monitoring their own speech, as well as hearing the other children when they spoke. (When I pointed this out to one principal who was taking me for a tour of the school, her response floored me. She said, and I quote, "It is against school policy for the children to hear themselves when they speak.") As far as loop systems are concerned, the hearing aids at the time did not include a microphone/telephone position, so that auditory self-monitoring was impossible. With a personal FM system, on the other hand, because of the location of the microphone, the children could consistently receive the teacher's speech at a high S/N ratio. And when the FM receivers later incorporated an environmental microphone, the children could also effectively monitor their own speech, as well as hear the other children to some extent.

While these conclusions are obvious now, they were not well accepted at first by educators, administrators, and audiologists and speech-language pathologists. Administrators in particular were very hesitant about approving money to purchase what they thought was an experimental system; they demanded evidence of its efficacy. This hesitation led Tom Giolas and me to try to provide such proof with several studies that we undertook (Ross & Giolas, 1971; Ross, Giolas, & Carver, 1973). What we did was compare PBK scores of children who were hard of hearing with and without their use of a personal FM system. The studies were conducted in a typical classroom and the children listened to the words the way they usually did, that is, either monaurally or binaurally and with either body or BTE hearing aids. Our purpose was very practical and focused: we wanted to know if—and if so, how much—word discrimination scores (auditory access) could be improved when the children used a personal FM system compared with their usual practice of listening to the classroom teacher.

We found the results to be rather astounding: the children's word discrimination scores typically doubled or tripled when they used a personal FM system compared with their usual mode of hearing the teacher. Even though these were rather primitive studies by modern standards, they have not to my knowledge been seriously refuted; the positive educational-clinical implications still hold. If children are to learn in classrooms, they must be able to hear the teacher as well as possible; this is exactly what any sort of classroom amplification system is designed to do. Unfortunately, it took many years for the implications of these research results to be translated into the routine use of such systems in classrooms. I would attribute much of this reluctance to provide listening systems (of all kinds) to the tendency of normally hearing people to judge the acoustical acceptability of a classroom setting by using the evidence of their own ears. Because they may have little or no difficulty in comprehending speech in that setting, it is hard for them to fully appreciate the deleterious effect that the acoustical conditions can have on someone with a hearing loss.

Research results, such as the studies conducted by Tom Giolas and myself, may have helped somewhat, but actually replicating the auditory experience of children with hearing loss in classrooms (or adults in some large venue) was even more convincing. We had to have some way (and I think we still do) to give normal hearing people some taste of the acoustical challenges faced daily by children with hearing loss in classrooms. One activity I undertook—with the help of graduate students including, as I recall, the co-editor of this book, Joe Smaldino—to achieve this goal was to remove a child's hearing aid from his or her ear and record the teacher's voice through a portable coupler to represent the way it would have been delivered to the child. Playing this back to the teacher (and school administrators) was a very convincing argument for the use of a personal FM system. We did this with parents, too, but stopped when the experience proved too emotionally devastating for them.

Too often, the signal emerging from the hearing aid was distorted beyond recognition; while the parents may not have been technically proficient, they could easily recognize the impossible acoustic challenge their children faced. These parents and teachers became "believers" (for a little while anyway). Indeed, in my judgment, the greatest challenge confronting the profession, in terms of the effects that poor room acoustics (and microphone technique) can have upon the auditory access of people with hearing loss, is sensitizing the normal hearing public to these effects. Without full appreciation of the consequences of poor acoustical conditions, those people responsible for allocating the necessary funds to purchase assistive listening systems and acoustically treating a classroom would be reluctant to do so.

◆ Acoustic Access for Adults

Even though the focus of this book is on school children in classrooms, a few words regarding auditory access for adults may be useful (these kids will grow up, after all). The same need that children have for an improved S/N ratio applies to adults with hearing loss who are listening in large spaces (auditoriums, theaters, houses of worship, etc.). I doubt that any audiologist reading these words has not heard clients bitterly complain about their difficulty comprehending speech in such places. Still, from my perspective, the requirements of the ADA (Americans with Disability Act) to install listening systems in large-area listening venues has been something of a disappointment. It is not that they don't work; they work very well indeed. The difference such a system can make, as I can personally attest, is simply astounding.

Years ago, a graduate student and I (Bankoski & Ross, 1984) compared the word recognition scores that an adult group achieved with and without a large-area FM system. We found, as with personal FM systems, that word recognition scores generally improved by 100 or 200 percent. The problem with these systems is not how they work, but rather that they are woefully neglected by those most in need of such systems. Theater and movie house managers complain that few people take advantage of the expensive listening systems that they installed. In other words, the technology is available; now it is necessary for audiologists to inform their clients about the existence of large-area listening systems and to encourage them to try using these systems. It is not just a professional responsibility; the end user—the person with a hearing loss—must leave his or her comfort zone and demand that large-area public venues provide such systems, in accordance with the law. And then they must actually use them. (The reasons people don't take advantage of the availability of listening systems merits a chapter in its own right.)

◆ Hearing Aids and Acoustic Access

This brings up the final link in the signal delivery chain: the characteristics of the sound entering one's ear canal. No matter how favorable the earlier links in the signal transmission may be (say, a reverberation time of 0.6 second and an ambient noise level of 35–40 dBA), if the sound is being perceived through a faulty hearing aid, or one fit improperly, this defeats our efforts to provide an optimal auditory-verbal signal to a listener who experiences a hearing loss. Many years ago, Gaeth and Lounsbury (1966) found that only 16 percent of the hearing aids worn by elementary school–age children could be considered completely adequate. This considered only the aid itself, not how well the hearing aid met the specific amplification needs of a child. Add deleterious classroom acoustics to this deplorable record and one can understand why so many children with hearing loss performed so poorly in schools.

Undoubtedly, the situation has improved considerably since those early days. Physically and electroacoustically it certainly has. Modern hearing aids have little in common with the hearing aids of the early days, other than the fact that they both amplify sounds. Nevertheless, one can question if present-day children, even in the best acoustical circumstances, are being provided hearing aids that optimally compensate for their specific hearing loss. Such pessimism is based on the fact that only a minority of audiologists use real-ear measures to fit and verify the fitting of a hearing aid. Until this final link in the signal delivery chain can be ensured, we can question whether the best possible auditory access has been achieved.

In brief, auditory access is a multifaceted concept. This book focuses on the acoustic challenge facing children in classrooms, a crucial topic that deserves as much treatment as it can get, but the larger goal is ensuring that an optimal auditory signal is being delivered to those who need it the most. What is at stake is not just sound, but a vital bridge to these people's future, to help them become productive members of our society.

References

Bankoski, S. M., & Ross, M. (1984). FM systems' effect on speech discrimination in an auditorium. *Hearing Instruments, 35*, 8–12.

Gaeth, J. H., & Lounsbury, E. (1966, August). Hearing aids and children in elementary schools. *Journal of Speech and Hearing Disorders, 31*(3), 283–289.

Ross, M. (1972). Classroom acoustics and speech intelligibility. In J. Katz (Ed.), *Handbook of clinical audiology.* Baltimore, MD: Williams and Wilkins.

Ross, M., & Giolas, T. G. (1971, December). Effect of three classroom listening conditions on speech intelligibility. *American Annals of the Deaf, 116*(6), 580–584.

Ross, M., Giolas, T., & Carver, P. W. (1973). The effect of classroom conditions on speech intelligibility: A replication in part. *Language, Speech, and Hearing Services in Schools, 4,* 72–76.

2

Hearing Is the Foundation of Listening and Listening Is the Foundation of Learning

Douglas L. Beck and Carol Flexer

◆ Introduction

Known and Unknown: A Memoir is the title of a 2011 book by Donald Rumsfeld. Politics aside, the premise of the title is that there are things we know, there are things we don't know but that we are aware of, and—digging deeper—there are important things that, frankly, we don't know and we are not aware of. Rumsfeld refers to these three categories (respectively) as "known knowns," "known unknowns" and "unknown unknowns." In communication disorders (admittedly a universe somewhat distant from politics) these three categories are also of importance.

For example, we know we are very likely accurate when we discuss tympanograms, auditory brainstem response (ABR), acoustic reflexes, and otoacoustic emissions (OAEs). In Rumsfeld's terms, these clear and objective measures of auditory phenomena, grounded more or less in indisputable facts, might be considered "known knowns." Of course, there are things we don't necessarily know with respect to each child or adult, yet we are aware of their importance. Such "known unknowns" might include ear canal resonance, outer and inner hair cell population integrity, possibly speech-in-noise ability, and perhaps how closely a specific hearing aid fitting approximates the real-ear "target." Taking the analogy to completion within the communication disorders universe, "unknown unknowns" might include processing speed, auditory processing disorders, listening skills, working memory, and attention—all of which significantly impact the child's listening ability and ultimately the child's learning ability.

The purpose of this chapter is to discuss the neurological and experiential basis of hearing, listening, and learning as impacted by acoustic accessibility in children and adults.

◆ Hearing and Listening

Audiologists generally measure hearing. Specifically, audiologists tend to measure "objective" and sensory-based percepts of pure tones, beeps, clicks, words, phonemes, and more. These test protocols effectively approximate human hearing acuity and help reveal the gross status of the peripheral auditory nervous system with respect to the stimuli used. However, and significantly, these measures do not reflect our formative ability to listen.

Frankly, there is much more to listening than hearing. For humans, the ability to listen is one of the many cognitive processes that separates us from all other animals, including those whose hearing is superior to that of humans. Indeed, "listening is where hearing meets brain" (Beck & Flexer, 2011). Beck and Flexer (2011) noted that dogs have much better hearing (perhaps 50 to 40,000 Hz) than humans (generally stated as 20 to 20,000 Hz). If cognition and learning were actually based on hearing, dogs (and cats, dolphins, whales, and many other animals) would be way above humans on the food chain. They are not. Dogs hear better than we do, but they cannot actually listen. For example, some dogs work tirelessly for years and years to learn to obey the command "sit." Their performance really is not about hearing; their performance is all about listening. (And don't get us started on cats.) Specifically, although hearing is the means through which sound reaches the brain, listening is what separates people from all other beings.

Humans with normal hearing and normal cognitive ability learn to listen. That is, humans apply meaning, context, concepts, ideas, thoughts, and more to spoken (and written) words to communicate and share ideas and concepts and to travel backward and forward across time and space. Our words and listening skills allow us to describe things beyond the here and now. We can describe things we have never seen, and we can even describe sounds we have never heard.

The task of normally functioning ears and hearing systems is to transmit acoustic information to the brain. However, hearing is a sense and hearing is passive. Listening is a learned skill and listening is active. At the moment speech sounds are perceived by the brain, listening occurs, and the skills of the listener are of significant importance. When hearing meets brain, "listening" occurs (Beck & Flexer, 2011); that is, we hear with our brains! Unfortunately (or perhaps fortunately), measuring the sensory capacity of a particular person to hear sounds (as represented on an audiogram) is just a small fraction of what matters (i.e., listening). Active listening is very much the same thing as "paying attention," and paying attention (and the ability to pay attention) is of critical importance with regard to listening and cognition.

◆ Auditory Processing Disorders

Quite simply, the whole concept of auditory processing disorders in children (and in adults too) remains highly controversial. The exact relationship between hearing, listening, auditory processing, auditory processing disorders (APD), attention, working memory and learning remains elusive. In fact, Kamhi (2011) wrote that APD "is best viewed as a processing deficit that may occur with various developmental disorders" (p. 270). Moore (2011) stated that the problem and the solution in relation to APD may well revolve around auditory cognition—with an emphasis on working memory and attention. Indeed, Moore and colleagues reasoned that when a child performs poorly on a traditional APD test, one should expect the child to demonstrate impaired listening ability. However, APD testing relies on cognitive and sensory abilities, and Moore states that the most common reason children present with poor listening skills appears to be impaired memory and attention-related issues. Although Lucker (2007) noted, "To date, we have not reached a consensus as to how we define, describe, evaluate and manage children with APD problems," more recently Moore, Cowan, Riley, Edmondson-Jones, and Ferguson (2011) reported a general lack of scientific rigor and testable hypotheses with regard to APD tests and a "bewildering array of tests, the majority of which lack any scientific basis or clearly defined clinical utility."

◆ Paying Attention

Richtel (2010) reported Strayer's observation that "attention is the Holy Grail." In response, Beck (2010) commented, "Where you attend is how you will do." Attention is finite. Indeed, when one divides one's attention, that is, multitasks, neither task is performed maximally. This is particularly true with regard to cognitively demanding tasks such as driving an automobile and simultaneously texting! Recently, the National Highway Traffic Safety Administration (NHTSA, 2005) reported that 80 percent of all car crashes involve a driver distraction within three seconds of the crash.

Ashcraft and Klein (2011) recently stated that "attention is a process that involves a finite commodity." Craik (2007) reported that outcomes with respect to hearing aid amplification are generally dependent on the allocation of attentional processes. Again, where you pay attention "is how you will do."

◆ Working Memory

Working memory is more or less what we used to refer to as "short term memory . . . typically no longer than 30 seconds." The term "short term memory" has been judged essentially inadequate with regard to defining its role in cognition and has been replaced (for more than a decade) with the term "working memory" (WM). WM allows us just enough time to rehearse the material or perform some other mental operations on the material. Boudreau and Costanza-Smith (2011) note WM impacts a vast quantity of cognitive processes, including learning rate for new vocabulary, language comprehension, literacy skills, reasoning, and problem solving, as well as overall academic success. Further, they state that WM controls attention and information processing.

◆ Bottom-up and Top-down Systems

Many of these issues (and related ones) have been discussed in the audiology and hearing aid literature using the terms "bottom-up" (to represent sensory information transmitted from the peripheral auditory nervous system to the brain) and "top-down" (to represent how the brain interprets the perceived acoustic information). Beck and Clark (2009) stated that when bottom-up and top-down systems function optimally, "precise and extraordinary meaning" is extracted from the "cacophony of sounds" in the acoustic environment—and this occurs virtually without effort. They report humans are unique in their ability to "apply cognitive processes (knowledge, memory, attention, and intelligence) to sensory input, to communicate, to learn, and to share thoughts and ideas."

Madell (2009) reports that audiologic measures of physiological events (ABR, ASSR, OAEs) are highly correlated with hearing, but cautions that they are not direct measures of hearing and, further, that people (i.e., children) with hearing loss have damaged auditory systems. People with hearing loss cannot achieve maximal auditory competence without specific training and, of note, even with appropriate amplification they need to learn to listen and to maximally use auditory information. Children taught to maximize their auditory skills develop significantly better speech and language skills than those who do not undergo auditory habilitation and rehabilitation (Osmond, 2011).

◆ Aural Rehabilitation: Not Just for Kids

When listeners have been trained to maximally employ the bottom-up (sensory-based) stimuli available to them, extraordinary things have occurred.

Gordon-Salant and Friedman (2011) reported a particularly illustrative example with regard to 10 older blind adults, 60 through 80 years of age, compared with two groups of 10 normally sighted younger (ages 18 through 30 years) and older (ages 60 through 80 years) adults. Using 40 to 60 percent time-compressed speech as a rather challenging listening task, the authors reported the blind adults recognized time-compressed speech better than their age-matched peers, and indeed, the blind adults performed similarly to the much younger, sighted adults. Of note, 8 of the 10 blind adult participants had trained themselves via time-compressed "books on tape" recordings to maximize their listening skills through motivated, dedicated, and conscious practice. Specifically, hearing is a sense and listening is a skill—and skills can be taught to help compensate for sensory deficits (i.e., blindness) and to help improve listening ("where you attend is how you will do").

Martin (2007) presented interesting observational data based on hundreds of patients fitted with hearing aids. One hundred and seventy-three of her hearing aid patients were given a software-based aural rehabilitation (AR) program (Listening and Communication Enhancement, LACE); 452 hearing aid patients were not given the software. In general, the LACE program requires a total time commitment of 10 hours over a 30-day period. Of the patients who underwent AR training, only 3.5 percent returned their hearing aids. Of those who had no AR training, 13.1 percent returned their hearing aids. Martin reports that statistical analysis revealed the only variable in the two groups was the AR training. One possible interpretation of these data is that patients trained in listening skills were better able to successfully employ hearing aids.

Stacey and colleagues (2010) reported on the effectiveness of a computer-based, self-administered AR training program for adult users of cochlear implants (CIs). Despite each of the 11 adults having worn the CI for at least three years, after a total AR training period of only 15 hours, a statistically significant increase in consonant perception was recorded.

Akeroyd (2008) reported that when facing acoustically challenging situations, such as hearing amid noise, adult listeners depend on previously acquired knowledge to "fill in the blanks." Specifically, when hearing loss prevents the entire acoustic image from being perceived at the sensory level, by definition, a degraded auditory signal is transmitted to the brain. For adults with good to excellent cognitive abilities, the missing components of the auditory signal are often resolved via top-down (i.e., cognitive) processes. Pichora-Fuller (2008) notes that cognitive ability, working memory, and vocabulary are indeed closely related to successful hearing aid use. That is, people with the most able cognitive systems tend to do best with processing auditory information.

Rawool (2007) notes that to accurately perceive rapid speech, listeners must attend to the signal while dividing their attention between monitoring the ongoing speech and actively applying cognitive processes to make sense of the acoustic information.

◆ Hearing Is the Foundation of Listening and Listening Is the Foundation of Learning

With specific regard to children and education, Flexer (2005) reported hearing is of paramount concern. She stated that when a child cannot clearly and easily hear spoken instruction (from the teacher, e.g.), "the entire premise of the educational system is undermined." Further, she states that *most* of what children learn about language and societal rules occurs through "passive" or "incidental" listening. Beck and Clark (2009) reported that one cannot process that which is not perceived. That is, hearing "drives" the entire process, and fortunately (Beck & Flexer, 2011) "any child with any degree of hearing loss can receive sound through one or more modern and advanced hearing access technologies."

The amount of practice required for continually wiring and rewiring the brain for higher-order language skills and the acquisition of knowledge is enormous. Gladwell (2008), Levitin (2006), and others report 10,000 hours of practice is needed for one to become an expert in a particular skill. Hart and Risley (1999; 2003) report that, by the age of 4 years, typical children need to have heard 46 million words to be ready for school. Dehaene (2009) reports 20,000 hours of listening are necessary in infancy and early childhood as a basis for reading.

Implications for Children

Indeed, if the bottom-up signal is missing, distorted, or impoverished (due to noisy classrooms, for example), the top-down system must work harder to make sense of the acoustic information (Allen et al., 2003). For children, filling in the blanks (a top-down process) is a remarkably difficult task because children require a very high signal-to-noise ratio to perform as well as adults with respect to acoustics. Further, and of enormous importance, children do not have advanced knowledge as to how conversations are likely to unfold, nor do they have the vocabulary required to "fill in the blanks." In addition, their ability to predict conversational twists and turns is much less than that of a mature adult.

◆ Summary

Typical mainstream classrooms are auditory-verbal environments where instruction is presented through the teacher's spoken communication. Children in a mainstream classroom, whether or not they have a hearing loss, must be able to hear, attend to, and listen to the teacher and each other in order for learning to occur. If the brains of children cannot consistently and clearly receive spoken instruction, the major premise of the educational system is undermined. This is what "acoustic accessibility" is all about.

Acoustic accessibility is critical because in environments relying on spoken language instruction, sounds have to reach the brain—the bottom-up feature—in order for learning to occur—the top-down feature. Therefore, we need to consider the environment of the classroom to enable us to provide the brain access to spoken instruction. The following chapters in this text will discuss the details of speech perception, room acoustics, and the use and efficacy of classroom audio distribution systems (CADS) as ways of understanding and managing the classroom learning environment.

References

Akeroyd, M. A. (2008). Are individual differences in speech reception related to individual differences in cognitive ability? A survey of 20 experimental studies with normal and hearing impaired adults. *International Journal of Audiology, 47*(Suppl. 2), S125–S143.

Allen, N. H., Burns, A., Newton, V., Hickson, F., Ramsden, R., Rogers, J., et al. (2003, March). The effects of improving hearing in dementia. *Age and Ageing, 32*(2), 189–193.

Ashcraft, M. A., & Klein, R. (2011). Attention. In D. J. Levitin (Ed.), *Foundations of cognitive psychology: Core readings* (2nd ed.). Boston, MA: Allyn and Bacon.

Beck, D. L. (2010). *Where you attend is how you will do.* Paper presented at the California Academy of Audiology (CAA) annual meeting, October 2010, San Francisco, CA.

Beck, D. L., & Clark, J. C. (2009, March/April). Audition matters more as cognition declines: Cognition matters more as audition declines. *Audiology Today* (American Academy of Audiology).

Beck, D. L., & Flexer, C. (2011, February). Listening is where hearing meets brain . . . in children and adults. *Hearing Review*. http://www.hearing review.com/issues/articles/2011-02_02.asp

Boudreau, D., & Costanza-Smith, A. (2011, April). Assessment and treatment of working memory deficits in school-age children: The role of the speech-language pathologist. *Language, Speech, and Hearing Services in Schools, 42*(2), 152–166.

Craik, F. I. M. (2007, July-August). The role of cognition in age-related hearing loss. *Journal of the American Academy of Audiology, 18*(7), 539–547.

Dehaene, S. (2009). *Reading in the brain: The science and evolution of a human invention.* New York, NY: Penguin Group.

Flexer, C. (2005). Rationale for the use of sound field systems in classrooms: The basis of teacher in-services. In C. C. Crandell, J. J. Smaldino, & C. Flexer (Eds.), *Sound field amplification: Application to speech perception and classroom acoustics* (2nd ed.). Clifton Park, NY: Delmar Cengage Learning.

Gladwell, M. (2008). *Outliers: The story of success.* New York, NY: Little, Brown.

Gordon-Salant, G., & Friedman, S. A. (2011, April). Recognition of rapid speech by blind and sighted older adults. *Journal of Speech, Language and Hearing Research, 54,* 622–631.

Hart, B., & Risley, T. R. (1999). *The social world of children learning to talk.* Baltimore, MD: Brookes.

Hart, B., & Risley, T. R. (2003). The early catastrophe: The 30 million word gap by age 3. http://www.aft.org/newspubs/periodicals/ae/spring2003/hart.cfm

Kamhi, A. G. (2011, July). What speech-language pathologists need to know about auditory processing disorder. *Language, Speech, and Hearing Services in Schools, 42*(3), 265–272.

Levitin, D. J. (2006*). This is your brain on music: The science of a human obsession.* New York: Plume Books.

Lucker, J. (2007). History of auditory processing disorders in children. In D. Geffner & D. Ross-Swain (Eds.), *Auditory processing disorders: assessment, management and treatment.* San Diego, CA: Plural Publishing.

Madell, J. R. (2009, March/April). The challenges ahead in pediatric audiology. *ENT and Audio News, 18*(1), 66–68.

Martin, M. (2007, August). Software-based auditory training program found to reduce hearing aid return rate. *Hearing Journal, 60*(8), 32–35.

Moore, D. R. (2011, July). The diagnosis and management of auditory processing disorder. *Language, Speech and Hearing Services in Schools, 42*, 303–308.

Moore, D. R., Cowan, J. A., Riley, A., Edmondson-Jones, A. M., & Ferguson, M. A. (2011, May-June). Development of auditory processing in 6- to 11-yr-old children. *Ear and Hearing, 32*(3), 269–285.

NHTSA. (2005). http://vtrc.virginiadot.org/Contact.aspx

Osmond, J. (2011). Interview. http://www.audiology.org/news/Pages/20110815.aspx

Pichora-Fuller, M. K. (2008, August). Audition and cognition: Where the lab meets clinic. *ASHA Leader, 13*(10), 14–17.

Rawool, V. W. (2007, September). The aging auditory system, part 3: Slower processing, cognition and speech recognition. *Hearing Review.*

Richtel, M. (2010, August 15). Outdoors and out of reach, studying the brain. *New York Times.* http://www.nytimes.com/2010/08/16/technology/16brain.html

Rumsfeld, D. (2011). *Known and unknown: A memoir.* New York, NY: Penguin Group.

Stacey, P. C., Raine, C. H., O'Donoghue, G. M., Tapper, L., Twomey, T., & Summerfield, A. Q. (2010, May). Effectiveness of computer-based auditory training for adult users of cochlear implants. *International Journal of Audiology, 49*(5), 347–356.

3 Speech Perception in the Classroom

Arthur Boothroyd

◆ Acoustics and Learning

We begin with two assumptions. First, classrooms are intended for learning. Second, much of that learning is mediated by speech. If these assumptions are correct, it follows that students in a classroom need to hear speech clearly—both the speech of the teacher and the speech of other students. But the amount of information in a talker's speech that actually reaches the ear of a listener depends on the acoustic properties of the room (Boothroyd, 2004; Nabelek & Nabelek, 1994; Yacullo & Hawkins, 1987). To put it simply, poor acoustics undermine the very purpose for which the classroom was intended.

◆ Clear Hearing

Perfectly clear hearing for speech may be defined as audibility of all the useful information in the acoustic speech signal. In other words, clear hearing is achieved when 100 percent of the information in the sound leaving the talker's mouth is present in the sound arriving at the listener's ear. One of the factors affecting audibility is the wide range of amplitude levels among speech sounds. By way of illustration, think of the decibel (dB) as if it were a measure of height. **Figure 3.1** shows a "speech elf" who is 30 dB high. The loud vowel sounds in speech (for example, *oo* and *aw*) are at the level of his hat, and the weak consonant sounds (for example, *f* and *th*) are at the level of his shoes. The average height of his clothing is 15 dB, at the level of his belt. If we think of room acoustics as a river he must cross as he travels from talker to listener, the goal of clear hearing is not just to keep his head above water, but also to keep his feet dry.[1]

Perfectly clear hearing is difficult to achieve. Fortunately, however, spoken language is highly redundant. In other words, the

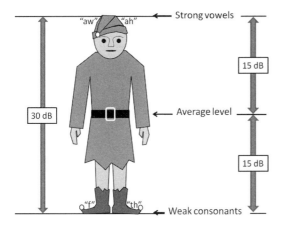

Fig. 3.1   If we think of the decibel as the unit of height of a "speech elf," and we think of the room as a river to be crossed, our goal is to keep his feet dry as he travels from talker to listener.

spoken language contains more information than the listener actually needs to understand the messages it carries. It is generally assumed, for example that adults can function adequately when only around 50 to 60 percent of the useful information in the speech sounds is available. This, however, requires that the listener takes full advantage of his or her mature knowledge and processing skills, and the listener may expend considerable mental effort in making up for the missing acoustic information. In addition, performance will break down if the language becomes complex and unfamiliar. Casual conversation may be possible in a noisy restaurant, but following a serious lecture, with the same level of noise in the background, can be virtually impossible.

There are many reasons to assume that children in a classroom need to receive much more than 60 percent of the useful information carried by the sounds of speech. First, they do not have the mature world, social, and language knowledge to enable them to take full advantage of context. Second, they do not have the mature speech processing skills that might enable them to keep pace with the talker while absorbing the meaning of what is being said. Third, much of the language used in a classroom is unfamiliar; that is, after all, the nature of a learning environment. It is not easy to determine the lowest level of information transmission consistent with optimal learning, and this almost certainly differs from child to child. For present purposes, however, let us assume something in the range of 90 to 100 percent as a working target.

◆ Enemies of Clear Hearing

Distance

There are three main enemies of clear hearing. The first is distance. As speech sound travels away from the talker it loses 6 dB of amplitude for every doubling of distance. As an example of the 6 dB rule, think of the speech produced by a Greek actor in an open-air amphitheater. A listener who is standing at a distance of, say, 10 feet (roughly 3 m) might hear the actor's speech at an average level of 56 dB SPL.[2] But a listener at a distance of 20 feet would hear it at a level of only 50 dB SPL, and a listener at a distance of 40 feet would hear it at a level of 44 dB SPL, as illustrated in **Fig. 3.2**.

If we put our Greek actor and his audience into a classroom, things get a little different. The listener hears not only the speech coming directly from the talker but also speech that is reflected from the room's surfaces. The 6 dB rule applies up to a certain distance, but beyond this *critical distance* (see below) the level is de-

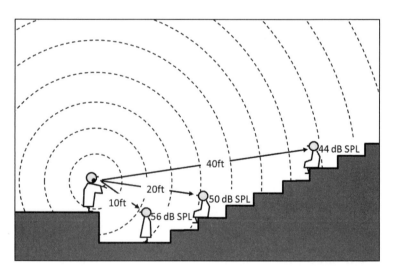

Fig. 3.2 Speech going directly from talker to listener loses 6 dB for every doubling of distance traveled.

termined mainly by reflected sound and remains fairly constant in spite of increasing distance, as illustrated in **Fig. 3.3**.

For a listener who is relying on sound reflections, the increased level is helpful. In **Fig. 3.3**, for example, the most distant of the three listeners receives the speech at a level that is some 6 dB above what he would experience without the reflections. As we shall see in a moment, however, this increase in decibel level from reflected sound comes at a cost.

Noise

The second enemy of clear hearing is noise. In the present context, noise refers to any sound that interferes with what the listener needs to hear. Some noises are generated outside the classroom. They pass through (or around) walls, doors, and windows. Sometimes they are carried into the room by the building's structure. Other noises are generated inside the classroom. They come from such things as air conditioners, fans, aquarium pumps, chairs (when they scrape the floor), footsteps, and, of course, the students themselves.

Noise obscures, or *masks*, some of the speech sounds, thereby reducing audibility. To avoid this, the average level of the speech

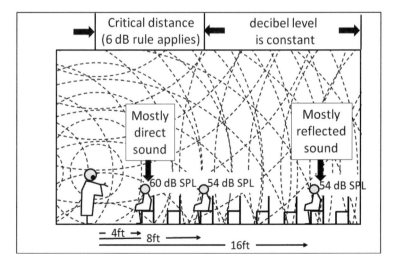

Fig. 3.3 Listeners at the back of a room enjoy an increase of speech amplitude because of multiple reflections from the room's boundaries.

needs to be at least 15 dB above that of the noise. If this criterion is met, one can assume that audibility is not reduced by noise. In other words, the listener can hear the weakest sounds in the speech signal. Another way of expressing this criterion is that the speech-to-noise ratio needs to be at least +15 dB. In **Fig. 3.4**, we use our speech elf to illustrate what happens to audibility as the speech-to-noise ratio falls from +15 dB (giving clear hearing) to −15 dB (giving no hearing at all). You will see that, when the levels of the speech and the noise are the same, the speech-to-noise ratio is 0 dB, giving 50 percent audibility of the useful information in the speech signal.[3]

Consider our theatergoers from **Fig. 3.1**, and imagine that there is a steady breeze blowing, creating a background noise with an average level of 29 dB SPL. As illustrated in **Fig. 3.5**, even the listener at 40 feet would still have full audibility of the actor's speech (44 dB SPL of speech minus the 15 dB criterion gives 29 dB SPL, which is the highest permissible noise level consistent with 100 percent audibility).

But now, in **Fig. 3.6**, consider the classroom and imagine a background noise level of 50 dB SPL (which is not unusual). Audibility for the nearest listener is 83 percent of what would be available in a quiet setting. This is already below our provisional criterion of 90 to 100 percent. The other two listeners receive only 63 percent

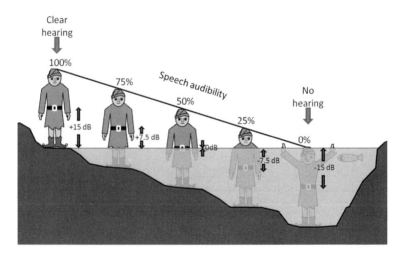

Fig. 3.4 Audibility of the useful information in the speech signal falls from 100 percent to 0 percent as the speech-to-noise ratio falls from +15 dB to −15 dB.

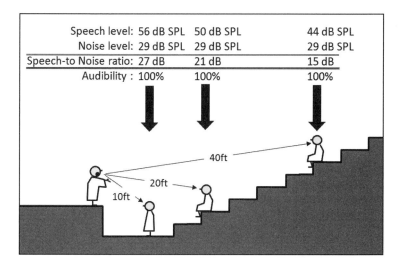

Fig. 3.5 With a 29 dB SPL noise background, created by a gentle breeze, all listeners enjoy a speech-to- noise ratio of 15 dB or more, allowing for 100 percent audibility of the useful information in the talker's speech.

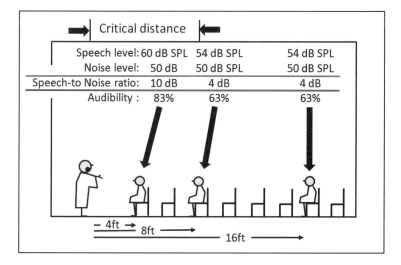

Fig. 3.6 With a 50 dB SPL noise background, created by both external and internal sources, no listener enjoys 100 percent audibility of the useful information in the talker's speech.

of the information they would receive in quiet. This is unacceptable. To eliminate the effect of noise for these two listeners would require that the noise level be reduced to 39 dB SPL.

In addition to preventing audibility of information in the speech signal, noise can be distracting. This is especially true if it carries potentially interesting information. Individuals differ in terms of their ability to ignore distractions and focus attention on a specific talker. There are, therefore, reasons other than speech audibility for controlling noise in a classroom. Distractible students may require a speech-to-noise ratio that is higher than 15 dB.

Reverberation

Definition

Reverberation is the persistence of sound in a room because of multiple, repeated reflections from the room's surfaces. At each reflection, some of the sound energy is absorbed, and the strength of the reflected sound is reduced. As a result, by the time it reaches the listener, the reflected sound is weaker than that traveling directly from the talker. There are so many reflections, however, that they add up to create a signal that is quite strong. In fact, as indicated earlier, there is a distance beyond which the total reflected sound is stronger than the direct sound. For a listener beyond this distance, the reflected sound determines the overall level of the speech signal at his or her ear.

Early and Late Reflections

Unfortunately, there is a potential downside to the reflected sounds. Because they have traveled a considerable distance, their arrival at the listener is delayed. If they arrive early enough after the direct sound (say, within one-twentieth of a second [50 milliseconds]), they add to the received level without undermining recognition (Bradley, Sato, & Picard, 2003). But if they arrive too late (say, after one-tenth of a second [100 milliseconds]), they cause an overlapping of speech segments (vowels and consonants) and recognition suffers (Nábělek, Letowski, & Tucker, 1989). The boundary between "early" and "late" is not easily defined but, as just suggested, is somewhere in the region of one-twentieth to one-tenth of a second (50 to 100 milliseconds). Speech is produced, on average, at a rate of around 13 vowels or consonants per second. This means that each sound, on average, is only ~75 milliseconds long. Delays greater than 75 milliseconds cause the sounds to run into each other excessively and the signal is degraded. Even if we attain a speech-to-noise ratio of 15 dB or more, we can no longer assume 100 percent audibility. Our speech elf may arrive with his feet dry, but he will be too tired to work as efficiently as we would like.

Reverberation Time

We measure the persistence of sound in a room in terms of the time it lasts. A room's *reverberation time* is the time it takes for the sound level to fall by 60 dB after the source stops. The abbreviation RT60 (or just RT) is used for this value. A reverberation time of 0.25 second will guarantee almost full clarity because the level of one sound will have dropped by 60 dB by the time the next sound is being heard. On the negative side, such a short reverberation time might deprive a distant listener of some of the benefits of reflected sound. In contrast, a reverberation time of 1 second could boost the speech level for a distant listener by 6 dB or more, but, because of late reflections, the information received may be below our 90 percent criterion. A reverberation time of around 0.5 second represents a reasonable compromise.

Critical Distance

As indicated earlier, *critical distance* refers to the distance beyond which reflected (or reverberant) sound dominates the speech level at a listener's ear. Listeners within the critical distance of the talker enjoy a signal that is clearer than do listeners who are beyond the critical distance.

Critical distance depends, in part, on reverberation time. For a small room that is 25 feet long, 25 feet wide, and 10 feet high (7.6 × 7.6 × 3 m) and that has a reverberation time of 1 second, the critical distance is around 5 feet (1.5 m), as shown at the top left in **Fig. 3.7**.[4] If we decrease the reverberation time to 0.25 second (a factor of 4), the critical distance doubles, as illustrated at the top right in **Fig. 3.7**. Note that the number of students within the critical distance from the teacher has increased from one to four.

Critical distance also doubles every time the room volume increases by a factor of 4. In a large room measuring 50 feet long by 50 feet wide (15 × 15 m), but with the same height of 10 feet (3 m) and a reverberation time of 1 second, the critical distance is around 10 feet (4 m), as shown in the bottom left portion of **Fig. 3.7**. De-

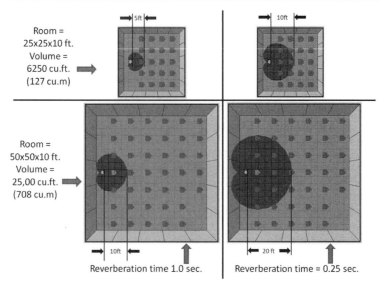

Fig. 3.7 The critical distance, shown here as the dark area around the teacher, increases as reverberation time decreases and as the size of the room increases.

creasing reverberation time of this room to 0.25 second doubles the critical distance to 20 feet, as illustrated at the bottom right portion of **Fig. 3.7**. In this case, the number of students within the critical distance from the teacher has increased from 3 to 10.

Figure 3.7 also illustrates the fact that the critical distance is greatest in front of the talker. The talker's head prevents the sound from being transmitted as effectively to the person's sides and back. The orientation of the talker, relative to the listener, is important.

◆ Interactions

The extent to which we benefit from addressing one enemy of clear hearing depends on the status of the other two. Consider, for example, the interdependence of noise and distance. As distance increases, speech level falls and the interfering effects of noise become more serious. Distance and reverberation also interact. Both the positive effects of early reflections and the negative effects of late reflections become more influential as the distance from talker to listener increases.

The interaction between reverberation and noise is less obvious but equally important. If the noise level is low, a distant listener can benefit from the additional clarity provided by a short reverberation time. To put this point in reverse terms, the benefits of reducing reverberation time can be squandered if noise is not also controlled.

◆ Factors Affecting Reverberation Time

Hard surfaces such as concrete, ceramic tile, plasterboard, glass, and varnished wood are efficient sound reflectors. The more such surfaces present in a room, the longer the reverberation time. There are surfaces, however, such as carpeting, acoustic tiles, curtains, upholstery, and clothing, that absorb most of the sound hitting them. The more these surfaces are present in a room, the lower the reverberation time.

Room size also affects reverberation time. In a large room the sound has to travel farther between reflections. As a result, it takes longer for sound to be absorbed at the reflecting surfaces.

◆ Frequency Effects

So far we have ignored the effects of frequency.[5] The sound patterns of speech contain many pure tones whose frequencies range from around 100 vibrations per second (Hz) to over 10,000 Hz. But useful information is not spread uniformly across this range. The highest concentration of information is in the region between 1000 and 4000 Hz (between two and four octaves above middle C on the piano). Similarly, noise covers a wide range of frequencies. The best guide to the interfering effects of noise is its amplitude in the range of 1000 to 4000 Hz. Finally, the reverberation time of a room is usually different at different frequencies. In assessing effects on speech reception, the reverberation time at 2000 Hz should be given priority.

◆ Reception and Recognition

The expression "useful information" has been used extensively in this chapter. Other terms for this concept are articulation index (ANSI, 1969; French & Steinberg, 1947; Kryter, 1962; Boothroyd,

2008), speech intelligibility index (ANSI, 1997), and speech transmission index (Steeneken & Houtgast, 1980). Each has its own definition but they all refer to the proportion, or percentage, of the useful information that a listener *receives*. What the listener *perceives* from this information is a different matter. Perception depends on a variety of factors, including the message's content and complexity, and the listener's attention, knowledge, and processing skill. Predicting speech *perception* from speech *reception* is difficult and involves many variables.

Figure 3.8 illustrates the combined effects of speech-to-noise ratio and reverberation time on one aspect of perception: the recognition of phonemes (vowel and consonants) in consonant-vowel-consonant (CVC) words.

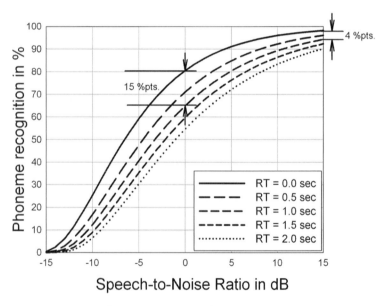

Fig. 3.8 Average phoneme recognition by young adults listening to consonant-vowel-consonant words presented in noise. Results are shown for speech that has been subjected to reverberation, with reverberation times from 0 to 2 seconds. The curves were derived by fitting hypothetical functions (Boothroyd, 2008) to data reported by Pegan (2007).

The results of Pegan's study suggest:

1. In the absence of reverberation, average phoneme recognition rises from 0 to 98 percent as the speech-to-noise ratio rises from −15 to +15 dB.

2. The degradation caused by reverberation reduces the useful information in the speech signal by around 12 percent per second of reverberation time (not visible in **Fig. 3.8**, but derived from the curve-fitting process).

3. At a speech-to-noise ratio of +15 dB, this loss of information results in a reduction of 4 percentage points in phoneme recognition per second of reverberation time (recognition drops from 98 to 94 percent).

4. At a speech-to-noise ratio of 0 dB (50 percent audibility), however, the loss of phoneme recognition increases to 15 percentage points per second of reverberation time (from 80 to 65 percent).

In a classroom setting, the effects of both noise and reverberation on speech perception are likely to be greater than is shown here because children have poorer vocabulary knowledge and processing skills than do adults. Nevertheless, these data serve to emphasize that the combined effect of noise and reverberation on the percentage of phoneme recognition is greater than the sum of their separate effects. The data also support the point made earlier—that management of classroom acoustics must address both noise and reverberation.

◆ Minimum Acoustic Requirements

Uncertainties about the varied acoustic needs of young children in real learning environments make it difficult to specify minimum acoustic requirements for classrooms. Indeed, a working group comprised of members from government, academia, and commerce spent four years arriving at the guidelines for classroom acoustics published by the American National Standards Institute (ANSI, 2002) (see subsequent chapters). In a small to medium-size classroom, these guidelines call for a maximum noise level of 35 dB SPL[6] and a maximum reverberation time of 0.6 second. The specifications are for an unoccupied room. Once the room is occupied, the reverberation time will be somewhat lower because of sound absorption by the children and their clothing. Unfortunately, the internally generated noise is likely to be higher. The goal behind these standards was to accept some degradation from reverberation but to attain at least a 15 dB speech-to-noise ratio for the least favorably situated student.

Consider the smaller of the two rooms illustrated in **Fig. 3.7**. Assume that it meets the ANSI guidelines when unoccupied but that, with the addition of 20 students and a teacher, the reverberation time at around 2000 Hz falls to 0.53 second. Assuming the talker's speech level at a distance of 1 foot (30 cm) to be 72 dB SPL, the predicted speech level at the back of the room is 56 dB SPL. A noise level of 35 dB SPL would then give a speech-to-noise ratio of 21 dB, which would satisfy the 15 dB criterion. It would also provide an additional 6 dB of "headroom" to allow for additional noise and the more stringent needs of young, distractible children. Based on the data from the previous section, the degradation introduced by reverberation would reduce the available information by around 6 percent, bringing the received information down to 94 percent. This value falls nicely within the range of 90 to 100 percent suggested earlier. (Note, again, that percent of information received and percent phoneme recognition are not the same thing.)

Things are also favorable for the larger of the two rooms in **Fig. 3.7**. Here, the ANSI guidelines allow for 0.7 second of reverberation time in acknowledgment of the technical difficulties of acoustic treatment in such a large space. With a teacher and 30 students, the reverberation time might drop to 0.66 second. Assume the teacher responds to the larger space by raising his speech level to 75 dB SPL at 1 foot. The predicted speech level received by a student at the back of the room is then around 54 dB SPL, and with a noise level of 35 dB SPL, the received speech-to-noise ratio is 19 dB. Once again, this meets the 15 dB criterion but with only 4 dB headroom. The reverberation would, however, cause an 8 percent reduction of information, bringing the received information down to 92 percent.

These calculations suggest that the ANSI guidelines, if followed, will produce classrooms that are suited to their intended function as learning environments in which speech is a primary mediator of that learning.

◆ What Can Be Done to a Bad Room?

It is an unfortunate fact of life that much teaching is done in classrooms that are acoustically hostile. There are, however, things that can be done in such situations.

Reverberation can be reduced by adding sound-absorbing materials to the room's surfaces. The addition of rugs, curtains, and carpet-lined cubbies can be helpful. If necessary, acoustic tiles can be placed on the ceiling and/or walls. Parallel reflecting surfaces should be avoided.

External noise can be kept out by eliminating spaces around doors and windows. Where possible, internal sources of noise should be removed (except for the students). One of the biggest offenders, however, is air circulation. Ventilation systems and heating/air conditioning vents create noise from turbulent air flow that is hard to eliminate.

One way to address residual noise is to increase the amplitude of the teacher's speech with a sound-field amplification system, also known as a Classroom Audio Distribution System (CADS). Speech is picked up by a microphone a few inches from the talker's mouth, where the speech-to-noise ratio is high and the contribution of reflections is negligible. This clear signal is then fed to strategically placed loudspeakers. Such systems are effective in increasing the speech-to-noise ratio for all students. The situation is analogous to providing our speech elf with stilts so that he can keep his feet dry as he crosses the river from talker to listener. Sound-field amplification systems also reduce the negative effects of reverberation for those students who are close to a loudspeaker. Sound-field amplification should not be used, however, as an excuse for poor management of noise and reverberation. More information on this topic can be found in later chapters of this book.

There are also things a teacher can do to minimize the effects of less-than-perfect room acoustics. Recommendations include (1) speak clearly and slowly to minimize the negative effects of reverberation (Payton, Uchanski, & Braida, 1994), (2) avoid talking with your back to the class, and (3) repeat the questions and answers of students for the benefit of the whole class. The third point is especially important when sound-field amplification is being used without a pass-around microphone.

◆ Summary

To fulfill their role as learning environments, classrooms should have acoustic properties that allow at least 90 percent of the useful information leaving a talker's mouth to reach the ears of all listeners. Factors working against this goal include distance, noise, and reverberation. Speech amplitude falls by 6 dB for every doubling of distance; noise masks the weaker sounds of speech; and, although the early components of reverberation can offset some of the effects of distance, the late components degrade the received signal. The goal of 90 percent audibility can be attained, however, if the speech-to-noise ratio for the most distant listener is 15 dB or more and if the reverberation time of the occupied room is in the region of 0.5 second. Appropriate guidelines satisfying these criteria have been published by the American National Standards Institute. In situations where the criteria cannot be met, the speech-to-noise ratio can be increased with the use of a sound-field amplification system. Sound-field amplification can also reduce the negative effects of reverberation for listeners who are close to a loudspeaker.

Notes

1. Note that the 30 dB range mentioned here does not take into account variations in average level between loud and soft talkers, or between loud and soft speech produced by the same talker. Adding these factors would increase the range to about 50 dB.
2. A decibel value tells us how much stronger one sound is than another. When referring to the average level of speech, we need to tell the reader what this level is being compared to. The standard reference is a very weak sound in which there are specified fluctuations of air pressure. In this case, we add the letters SPL (for sound pressure level) after "dB." Because they already represent differences, the 6 dB per doubling of distance and the 30 dB range between the louder and softer sounds in speech need no extension.
3. Note that the percentage of useful information is not the same as percent recognition. One is what the listener receives. The other is what he does with it. The relationship between the two depends on many factors. Some are related to the complexity of the language. Others are related to the knowledge and skill of the listener.
4. These and subsequent estimates use equations developed by Peutz (1997).
5. Changes of frequency in a sound pattern are heard as changes of pitch. Young adults, with normal hearing, can detect sounds whose frequencies fall in the range of 20 to 20,000 vibrations per second (Hz).
6. Actually 35 dBA. The "A" extension means that measurements are in SPL but with attenuation of low frequencies to more exactly reflect the characteristics of human hearing.

References

American National Standards Institute (ANSI). (1969). *American National Standard for calculation of the articulation index* (S3.5-1969). New York, NY: American National Standards Institute.

ANSI. (1997). *Methods for calculation of the speech intelligibility index* (S3.5-1997). New York, NY: American National Standards Institute.

ANSI. (2002). *Acoustical performance criteria, design requirements, and guidelines for classrooms* (S12.6-2002). New York, NY: American National Standards Institute.

Boothroyd, A. (2004). Room acoustics and speech perception. *Seminars in Hearing, 25,* 155–166.

Boothroyd, A. (2008, August). The performance/intensity function: An underused resource. *Ear and Hearing, 29*(4), 479–491.

Bradley, J. S., Sato, H., & Picard, M. (2003, June). On the importance of early reflections for speech in rooms. *Journal of the Acoustical Society of America, 113*(6), 3233–3244.

French, N. R., & Steinberg, J. C. (1947). Factors governing the intelligibility of speech sounds. *Journal of the Acoustical Society of America, 19,* 90–119.

Kryter, K. D. (1962). Validation of the articulation index. *Journal of the Acoustical Society of America, 34,* 1698–1702.

Nábĕlek, A. K., Letowski, T. R., & Tucker, F. M. (1989, October). Reverberant overlap and self-masking in consonant identification. *Journal of the Acoustical Society of America, 86*(4), 1259–1265.

Nábĕlek, A. K., & Nábĕlek, I. V. (1994). Room acoustics and speech perception. In J. Katz (Ed.), *Handbook of clinical audiology* (4th ed., pp. 624–637). Baltimore, MD: Williams and Wilkins.

Payton, K. L., Uchanski, R. M., & Braida, L. D. (1994, March). Intelligibility of conversational and clear speech in noise and reverberation for listeners with normal and impaired hearing. *Journal of the Acoustical Society of America, 95*(3), 1581–1592.

Pegan, K. (2007). Interactive effects of noise and reverberation on speech perception. (Unpublished AuD research thesis). San Diego State University and University of California, San Diego.

Peutz, V. (1997). Speech reception and information. In D. Davis & C. Davis (Eds.), *Sound System Engineering* (2nd ed., pp. 639–644). Boston: Focal Press.

Steeneken, H. J. M., & Houtgast, T. (1980, January). A physical method for measuring speech-transmission quality. *Journal of the Acoustical Society of America, 67*(1), 318–326.

Yacullo, W. S., & Hawkins, D. B. (1987). Speech recognition in noise and reverberation by school-age children. *Audiology, 26*(4), 235–246.

4 Classroom Acoustic Measurements

Joseph J. Smaldino and Daniel Ostergren

◆ Introduction

A typical classroom is a dynamic environment that continually changes from one learning activity to another and as the spatial relationship between the speaker and listener varies. For this reason, acoustical environments of classrooms are often difficult to measure because acoustical parameters change as a function of time. For example, intensity variations in the teacher's voice and the background noise levels in the classroom continually alter the signal-to-noise (SNR) ratio. Therefore, a standardized understanding of the status and dynamics of a particular classroom must be understood before changes in the acoustical environment can be considered. Fortunately we have such standardization.

◆ Classroom Acoustic Standards

In recognition of the fact that undesirable acoustics can be a barrier to listening and learning in the classroom, a working group composed of a wide variety of stakeholders produced the first American standard, ANSI/ASA S12.60–2002, *Acoustical Performance Criteria, Design Requirements, and Guidelines for Schools* (ANSI/ASA, 2002). Since ANSI standards are reviewed on a regular cycle, another working group made up of a similar mix of stakeholders as the 2002 working group was formed to undertake the review. The working group considered revisions and debated public comments concerning the original standard. As a result of these debates and discussions, it was decided that a separate part should be devoted to issues unique to portable classrooms.

The first part of the revised standard, *American National Standard Acoustical Performance Criteria, Design Requirements, and Guidelines for Schools, Part 1: Permanent Schools* (ANSI/ASA, 2009/2010), is a refined version of the 2002 standard. The major performance requirement for furnished but unoccupied class-rooms is basically unchanged from the 2002 standard. The one-hour average A-weighted background noise level cannot exceed 35 dB (55 dB if C-weighting is used) and for average size classrooms (with a volume less than or equal to 10,000 cubic feet) the rever-beration time (RT60) cannot exceed 0.6 seconds (35/55 dBA/C and 0.7 seconds if the volume is greater than 10,000 but less than or equal to 20,000 cubic feet). Among other changes are improvement of the requirements for exterior walls and roofs in noisy areas, consideration of activities close to classrooms, clarification of the definition of a "core learning space," addition of the limit of 45 dBA for sound in hallways, clarification and simplification of measure-ment procedures and addition of the requirement that, if an audio distribution system is deemed appropriate, it should provide even coverage and be adjustable so as not to disturb adjacent classes.

The second part of the revised standard, *American National Standard Acoustical Performance Criteria, Design Requirements, and Guidelines for Schools, Part 2: Relocatable Classroom Factors* (ANSI/ASA, 2009/2010), phases in performance requirements for portable classrooms. The current standard sets a 41 dBA limit for background noise in unoccupied classrooms, which would be lowered to 38 dBA in 2013 and 35 dBA in 2017. Reverberation time (RT60) in unoccupied relocatable classrooms must not ex-ceed 0.5 second in classrooms with volumes of 10,000 cubic feet or less and 0.6 second in classrooms with volumes of 10,000–20,000 cubic feet. Both parts of the standard are available with-out charge from the Acoustical Society of America store (http://asastore.aip.org).

A third part is currently under development and will focus on control of noise from informational technology in the classroom.

At this writing, compliance with the revised standards remains voluntary. Special effort was made during the crafting of the revi-sion to include language so that the standards could be considered for incorporation into the *International Building Code,* which would make compliance mandatory for new school construction. Efforts to incorporate the standards into the 2012 building code failed; an-other opportunity will occur when the International Code Council begins the 2015 building code development in 2013. As this Hand-book goes to press, the new ANSI classroom acoustics standards are being considered for inclusion in the revision of the *International Green Construction Code.* While final inclusion in the revised code (due sometime in 2011) is not a sure thing, it is a step in the right direction toward making acceptable classroom acoustics manda-tory in all classrooms.

◆ Screening for Compliance with ANSI Standards

The first step in determining if a classroom is in compliance with the ANSI acoustic standards is to complete a preliminary classroom acoustical survey. A survey worksheet is shown in Appendix 4.1. and is designed to be used by professionals with varying degrees of training and equipment. The purpose of the worksheet is to help identify classrooms that may have acoustical problems that interfere with communication and instruction. These problems affect a student's ability to attend, hear, listen, understand and participate in educational programs. These acoustical problems also will detract from the performance of a classroom audio distribution system (CADS) that might be in use. When noise and/or reverberation levels are suspected to exceed those recommended by ANSI/ASA S12.60 (ANSI/ASA, 2009/2010), the screening survey data are an indicator for further assessment. This assessment may include a referral to an acoustical specialist who can perform a comprehensive acoustical analysis and suggest solutions. Recall that the two performance criteria offered in the ANSI standards are background noise level and reverberation time (RT60). The following is a suggested method for conducting a preliminary classroom acoustical survey based on these criteria.

Directions for Classroom Background Noise Measurements (Section 1 of the Worksheet)

To conduct these measurements according to the ANSI standard, a Type 2 or better sound level meter (SLM) is required. It would be best to conduct the survey with an SLM that approximates this requirement. As you will see later in this chapter, it is possible to approach Type 2 accuracy using inexpensive hand-held devices. In addition, some sort of distance measuring device is required to construct an accurate schematic of the classroom situation. This measuring device can be as simple as a tape measure or may involve an inexpensive ultrasonic or laser distance-estimating device. The following directions refer to elements of the survey form found in Appendix 4.1:

1. Draw a schematic of the classroom on the back of the survey form or a separate piece of paper, marking the locations of the measurements (L1-L5). Generally, measurements should be taken from student desks at the four corners of the instruc-

tional area, the middle and the middle back of the room. If there is a target student, use location L1 to mark that student's position and eliminate middle back of room. Additional positions can be added if necessary.

2. Identify the make and model of the SLM used as well as the averaging timeframe. The ANSI/ASA S12.60 (ANSI/ASA, 2009/2010) standard requires a one hour average. When it is not possible to perform a one hour average, indicate, under the short-term option, the number of seconds or minutes and the number of time samples that were made to determine the average for each measurement (e.g., 5 time samples, 1 minute each). Type 2 SLMs may contain an averaging function to determine this value and often recommend a timeframe.

3. Sound level measurements should be taken in both A- and C-weighted conditions for the classroom background noise levels. A-weighting will capture a better estimate of speech information as received by the listener, while the C-weighting will focus on HVAC and other low-frequency noise in the classroom. If only one weighting is performed, select A-weighted.

4. Specific background noise measurement instructions are as follows:

   a. Turn on the SLM; set to the A- or C-weighted scale and slow response. If you can set the range of the meter, set it to accommodate 40–60 dB SPL to begin.

   b. Background noise levels should be measured for the unoccupied and occupied conditions at several locations in the classroom because levels may vary according to distance from noise sources. Indicate which condition you are using by circling the corresponding number (1=unoccupied, HVAC off; 2=unoccupied, HVAC on; 3=occupied, HVAC off; 4=occupied, HVAC on); use the column that corresponds to the weighting used for each of the measurements taken. Measure as many conditions as possible. When making short-term measurements, it is recommended that 3 to 5 one-minute time samples are averaged to determine the level. The ANSI/ASA S12.60 (ANSI/ASA, 2009/2010) standard is based on a one hour average unoccupied classroom with the HVAC on; therefore, a measurement in this condition is necessary when making a formal comparison to the standard.

   c. If the room is occupied, have the students remain quiet. Measure the background noise level at the selected student locations and record it on the worksheet. These measurements will provide an estimate of the background noise level during an instructional period. If measurements can only be taken in an empty classroom, you may estimate occupied classroom levels by converting the unoccupied noise levels to occupied by adding 10 dB to each unoccupied measurement. This conversion is comparable to reported differences in noise levels between *average* unoccupied and occupied classrooms (Bess et al., 1984; Sato & Bradley, 2008; Sanders, 1965).

d. Calculate and record the average background noise level for each condition measured. Compare with the ANSI/ASA S12.60 (ANSI/ASA, 2009/2010) standards for the weighting used and the size and type of room (permanent or portable).

Directions for Classroom Reverberation Measurements (Section 2 of the Worksheet)

Reverberation time (RT60) is defined as the amount of time in seconds that it takes a sound to decay by 60 dB in a room. RT60 can be measured in several ways. Some SLMs have the optional ability to determine RT60 and there are several computer-based software programs designed to directly measure reverberation using a variety of methods. Later in this chapter you will see how a smart phone can be used to determine this important classroom acoustic performance measure. Often, however, the RT60 is estimated using a formula and a paper-and-pencil methodology, based on absorption co-efficients of surface materials in a classroom. A brief description of each method follows and as before refers to the classroom acoustical survey form shown in Appendix 4.1.

Directions for RT60 Measurements

Equipment needed includes a reverberation time measuring instrument or sound level meter with reverberation time measurement capability, and a noise-generation source, such as a balloon or two boards that can be clapped together. Note: The following measurements should be made in empty classrooms for accuracy as well as to avoid exposure of occupants to loud noise:

1. Make separate RT60 measurements at 500 Hz, 1000 Hz and 2000 Hz.

2. These measurements require an impulse sound to be generated that is at least 25 dB louder than the background noise in the room. The impulse sound can be produced by dedicated sound generators, or more commonly, breaking balloons or slapping boards together.

3. Measurements at each frequency should be made in the four corners and the middle of the room. The five measurements at each frequency should be averaged to obtain the best estimate of the RT60 for that frequency in the room. Record this average on the form for each frequency. These locations can also be indicated on the classroom schematic.

4. An overall RT60 estimate in the classroom for the speech frequencies is obtained by averaging the RT60 estimates obtained for 500 Hz, 1000 Hz and 2000 Hz. Record this as the overall room average RT60.

Directions for Calculating Estimated RT60 Using the Sabine Formula

The most common formula for estimating reverberation time is the familiar Sabine equation (RT60 = .049 × Volume/Surface Area × Average Absorption). This equation can be used to make paper-and-pencil estimates of RT60.

Equipment needed includes a 20 foot measuring tape or ultrasound/laser distance measuring device, and a calculator.

Formula to estimate classroom reverberation time: RT = .049 × V/A where RT = reverberation time in seconds, V = volume room, and A = total absorption of the room surfaces in Sabins:

1. All of the reverberation estimates should be conducted in an unoccupied classroom. Because a formula is used, no improvement in accuracy is obtained with students and teacher present.

2. Calculate the volume of the classroom by measuring the length, width, and height of the classroom in feet and multiplying them together (volume = length of room × width of room × height of room). Some ultrasonic/laser measuring devices will perform this volume calculation after the initial measurements are made.

3. Record the resulting room volume in cubic feet on the classroom acoustical survey form.

4. Multiply the volume of the room by the constant 0.049 to obtain the numerator for the RT = .049 V/A equation. Record the results on the form.

5. To obtain the denominator of the equation, the area of the walls, floor, and ceiling of the room must first be calculated in square feet. Again the ultrasonic/laser measuring device may be able to determine the areas based on initial measurements. If the walls, ceiling, or floor is irregularly shaped, each section must be measured separately. The area of the floor and ceiling is determined by multiplying the length of the floor or ceiling times its width. The area of the walls can be obtained by multiplying the length of each wall by its height. Enter the values for the area of each on the classroom documentation form.

6. The absorption coefficient (ABS. Coef.) is a measure of the sound reflectiveness of different construction materials. The coefficient, expressed in Sabins, must be determined for the material composing the walls, ceiling, and floor. Average absorption coefficients are given in **Table 4.1** for the most common construction materials. If a different construction material is encountered and you use another absorption coefficient table, average the coefficients given in the other table for 500, 1000, and 2000 Hz for the purpose of these calculations. Enter the average absorption coefficient in the appropriate place on the survey form.

7. Multiply the area of each floor, ceiling, and wall times the absorptive coefficient of the material composing the surface (**Table 4.1**). Add up all of the resultants of the multiplications to obtain the A (total absorption of the room in Sabins) in the RT = .049 V/A formula for the room and record it on the form.

8. Take the numerator from Step 3 (0.049 × V) and the denominator from Step 7 (A = total absorption in Sabins for the room) and divide them to determine the estimated reverberation time of the room in seconds (RT = .049 V/A). Enter the estimate on the documentation form. Compare the results to the ANSI/ASA S12.60 (2009/2010) standards for the type of room (permanent or portable).

Directions to Determine Approximate Critical Distance (Section 3 of Worksheet)

While critical distance is not an acoustic performance measure included in the current ANSI standard, the working group that revised the standard in 2009/2010 seriously considered adding

Table 4.1   Sound Absorption Coefficients for Common Classroom Materials[a]

Material	Average Absorbtion Coefficient
WALLS:	
Brick	0.04
Painted concrete	0.07
Window glass	0.12
Plaster on concrete	0.06
Plywood	0.12
Concrete block	0.33
FLOORS:	
Wood parquet on concrete	0.06
Linoleum	0.03
Carpet on concrete	0.37
Carpet on foam padding	0.63
CEILINGS:	
Plaster, gypsum, or lime on lath	0.05
Acoustical tiles (5/8″)–suspended	0.68
Acoustical tiles (1/2″)–suspended	0.66
Acoustical tiles (1/2″)–not suspended	0.67
High absorptive panels–suspended	0.91

[a]Adapted from Berg, F. S. (1993) (p. 78). In C. C. Crandell, J. J. Smaldino, & C. Flexer (Eds.), *Sound-field FM Amplification*. San Diego, CA: Singular Publishing Group (1995). Reprinted by permission. See RT60 Web sites for a more comprehensive list of materials.

it. Critical distance demarcates the distance from a sound source when the direct (no reverberation) and reverberant energy are equal. Since audiologists often recommend preferential seating in order for students to primarily receive direct sound, knowledge of the critical distance is helpful in making this sort of recommendation. Using **Table 4.2**, match the volume and estimated reverberation time of the room being analyzed. The resulting value is the critical distance. Up to and including this distance from the talker, reflections from the sound reverberating in the room will enhance the speech signal; beyond this distance, the speech signal will be degraded by the later reflections of the sound reverberations. For example, for a room of 10,000 cubic feet and a reverberation time of 0.4 seconds, the critical distance is 10 feet. It is important that students with special listening requirements are not positioned any further than 10 feet from the talker in this situation to receive the most intelligible signal from the talker.

Table 4.2 Estimated Critical Distance Table[b]

Room Volume (cubic ft.)	Reverberation Time (seconds)							
	.3	.4	.5	.6	.7	.8	.9	1.0
2,000	5.2	4.5	4.0	3.7	3.4	3.2	3.0	2.8
4,000	7.3	6.3	5.7	5.2	4.8	4.5	4.2	4.0
6,000	8.9	7.7	6.9	6.3	5.9	5.5	5.2	4.9
8,000	10.3	8.9	8.0	7.3	6.8	6.3	6.0	5.7
10,000	11.5	10.0	8.9	8.2	7.6	7.1	6.7	6.3
12,000	12.6	11.0	9.8	8.9	8.3	7.7	7.3	6.9
14,000	13.7	11.8	10.6	9.7	8.9	8.4	7.9	7.5
16,000	14.6	12.6	11.3	10.3	9.6	8.9	8.4	8.0
18,000	15.5	13.4	12.0	11.0	10.1	9.5	8.9	8.5
20,000	16.3	14.1	12.6	11.5	10.7	10.0	9.4	8.9
	Critical Distance (feet)							

[b]© Arthur Boothroyd, used with permission.

◆ Classroom Acoustic Measurements: "The Times They Are a-Changin'"

While many audiologists daily survey classrooms for compliance with the ANSI performance criteria, many do not. The importance of desirable classroom acoustics for listening and learning in the classroom cannot be overstated and it behooves each and every audiologist to advocate for good acoustic environments in every classroom. Because some of the measurements just described require expensive instrumentation, many audiologists without this instrumentation have not been able to make the acoustic measurements needed to identify classrooms in need of strong advocacy for change or intervention. Well, "the times they are a-changin'" and technology has made it possible and inexpensive enough for each and every audiologist to be able to screen for classroom acoustic adequacy. The next section of this chapter will describe how this might be accomplished.

◆ There's an App for That

"There's an app for that!" There are few among us who have not either heard or uttered that phrase at some point over the last few years. The range and scope of applications for smart phones, tablets, and even laptops continue to grow at a rapid rate. In fact, since we are interested in applications for hand-held devices that are related to sound and sound measurement, should you need to judge a watermelon's ripeness, there's an app for that too! Simply hold your smart phone's microphone near the melon of interest and give it a thump—the melon that is. The app should let you know if it is ripe or not! While we have no experience with this application, it may be the most unusual acoustical analysis application available. Perhaps you have found some others?

As amusing as a "melon meter" may be, we are interested in applying the sophisticated and evolving technology available to us on our smart phones and other devices to issues far more important than the ripeness of a watermelon. We are interested in accurate, cost-effective, and easy-to-use approaches to measure the acoustical characteristics of classrooms. Specifically, as per the current ANSI standards, we would like to be able to accurately and reliably measure the unoccupied noise levels and octave band reverberation times that are present in a given classroom enclosure. Obtaining accurate data regarding these parameters allows us to document compliance (or lack of compliance) with the ANSI standard mentioned earlier in the chapter and affords us elegant tools with which to share this information with other stakeholders. It is critical to state that these measures cannot replace full acoustical analysis by certified acousticians, nor are they intended to do so. They are tools for audiologists to obtain and share essential information related to the acoustical challenges students face daily in their typical learning environments.

A recent online search of basic sound level meter apps available for Apple iOS and Android platforms yielded several that could be useful for the measurement of classroom acoustics. Of this small group, few appeared to have been designed by audio professionals for use by professionals, or could possibly be considered equivalent to stand-alone, Type 2 sound level meters (SLMs). The others seem to be designed more for estimation or amusement purposes only, lacking features such as A-weighting, spectral analysis, or measures of reverberation time, etc. While the options available may be limited, the well-designed apps can be extremely useful and may also be bundled with sophisticated features that go far beyond our area of interest. It should be noted that all apps from the silly to the sophisticated are simply manipulating and displaying data that have been input to the device either via the internet/cell phone service carrier (most games and other information delivery applications), or directly via the internal microphone, the headset input, or, in the case of Apple iOS devices, the 30-pin docking input—the place into which you connect the charger. Real-time, direct input is our area of interest, and a discussion of the advantages and limitations of the various direct input methods is warranted before examining specific measurement techniques, because the input method impacts the accuracy of our measurements, as we shall see. The following discussion is limited to Apple iOS devices (iPhone, iPod Touch, and iPad), because these devices, collectively, have the deepest market penetration. It is reasonable to assume that other platforms, such as Android, have similar characteristics.

The "weak link" in using an iPhone as an SLM or acoustic analyzer is the microphone, as the computing power in any of these devices is more than sufficient. The frequency response of the iPhone/iPad's built-in microphone, while quite consistent from unit to unit, has a steep low-frequency roll-off beginning at ~250 Hz of nearly 24 dB/octave. This low frequency roll-off minimizes wind noise when the phone is being used for its intended purpose, as a telephone. App designers must compensate for this feature and will generally state that low-frequency accuracy is somewhat compromised compared with accuracy at higher frequencies.

There are also external microphones that plug into the headset jack that claim to have greater accuracy than the built-in mic on the iPhone or iPad. While that may be true over all, the signal from *any* headset or external mic connected to the headphone jack must pass through the same filter set that the built-in mic does, thus producing the same 24 dB/octave low-frequency roll-off characteristic as the built-in mic. The microphone capsule itself may be more robust and linear than the built-in mic, but the low-frequency trade-off remains the same.

The next option is to use ancillary equipment that connects to the iPhone or iPad via the 30-pin docking connector. Interestingly, the docking connector on older devices, such as the iPhone 3GS, iPod Touch 3, and other models, was an analog-only input. This means that the conversion from an analog signal to a digital data stream suitable for analysis and manipulation was done inside the Apple iOS device. The quality of this conversion impacts the quality of the analysis, and while analog-to-digital converter (ADC) technology has reached a fairly mature state, smart phone manufacturers must manage costs appropriately, choosing ADCs that were perhaps not specifically designed for acoustical measurement purposes. Recent devices, such as the iPhone 4, iPod Touch 4, and iPad, have digital input docking connectors. This affords manufacturers of external hardware (and their dedicated software app) compatible with the Apple iOS to optimize the conversion process, thus ensuring that the device receives a suitable signal for analysis.

As you might imagine, moving from using the internal mic as a source to using a separate piece of hardware that houses a dedicated mic, ADC, and power supply adds cost. Purchasing a dedicated measurement mic from one manufacturer that interfaces with a quality piece of conversion/routing hardware from another, which in turn interfaces with an iPhone via the digital input of the docking connector, can approach the purchase price of a good Type 2 SLM. What's the point? There are two important points. First is flexibility. We can choose how deep we want to go with options, hardware, and applications. Some readers may wish to simply have an accurate SLM/reverberation analyzer at the ready on their smart phone. Others may wish to invest in other options allowing for more sophisticated measurement. Having options is great, as one may add features as needed. Second, and more importantly, is the ability to immediately share measurements with others. It is possible, with the right software, to actually have your measurements be displayed on another individual's phone in real time—amazing! More realistically, one can email a screen shot of the metric(s) of interest along with a short narrative explaining the results as a supplement to the full report. Summarizing and sharing data are therefore streamlined to the extreme. More regarding data sharing shortly.

So, where is an audiologist or other professional who is charged with documenting the acoustical properties of a classroom to start? Recall that most of the "negatives" of using an iPhone or iPad right out of the box in place of a dedicated piece of analysis hardware are related to two factors: having a well-designed app, and acknowledging that the built-in mic has limitations picking up sound energy below 250 Hz. Recall that dB A-weighting "ignores" low frequencies (as well as high-frequency extremes) somewhat compared with other frequencies in the audible range. In fact, a low-frequency roll-off of 10–20 dB below 250 Hz is noted when examining a dBA curve. Perhaps the on-board mic's frequency response variations are less serious than first thought. Frankly, the hardware contained in an off-the-shelf iPhone/iPad can conduct quite adequate acoustical measurements for our purposes.

Most important is whether the app one chooses provides a mechanism for calibration. Simply purchasing, downloading, and installing the app shouldn't imply that we're ready to go. Rather, it is necessary to conduct a comparative calibration using a reference SLM. From our experience, this can yield very good results. In fact, while assisting in the revision of a manufacturer's product recently, a calibrated smart phone was used as a cross-check SLM, and the readings typically differed by less than 1 dB from the development engineer's dedicated device, which costs thousands more. Nevertheless, one aspect of the built-in mic *is* a bit of an issue: We cannot couple it to a calibration device to document its accuracy and trim as needed. Comparing the iPhone's sound pressure level reading with that of a calibrated SLM while measuring a steady noise source, then trimming the calibration settings in the app's "settings" menu, is the only option. Instructions for calibrating the application should be available on the developer's Web site. By the way, where is the mic on an iPhone? It's on the *bottom.* Be mindful of how you are holding the device when using it as a measurement tool. For best results, hold it upside down. Where is the mic on an iPad? It's on the *top.* Hold the device accordingly.

On the other end of the spectrum, if one has the entire external mic/hardware system that interfaces with the iOS device via the 30-pin dock connector, it can be professionally calibrated and the procedure documented by the third party handling the task. You now have a true, Type 2 sound level meter with the additional capability of being able to send the results you've obtained anywhere you wish. (You also have an extraordinarily accurate "melon meter"!) While we would not hesitate to use measurements made by an Apple iOS device and app that has been carefully hand trimmed for reporting estimates of the acoustical properties of a classroom, such measurements would be inappropriate for research purposes or publication in a peer-reviewed journal. Only a professionally calibrated hybrid of smart phone/external mic and signal input system should be used in these instances.

Now that we are clear on some of the advantages and possible limitations of the gear, let's get down to the business of making some measurements! **Disclosure**: We currently use the AudioTools app bundle by Studio Six Digital. The developer is an audio professional, having manufactured several other high-quality stand-alone measurement systems. We use AudioTools on both the iPhone 4 and iPad 2. On the iPad, is used a MicW-i436 external mic. This mic is used because, as you can see in **Figs. 4.1** and **4.2**, the iPad is typically kept in a very sturdy case that unfortunately blocks the built-in mic port slightly. The external mic, plugged into the headset jack, allows the mic capsule to be outside of the case, as is apparent in both figures. Since we are not affiliated with Apple Computer, Studio Six Digital, or MicW corporations in any way, we encourage the reader to find hardware/software that best suits his or her needs.

Figure 4.1 shows an iPad 2 in its case, external mic connected (top right), with the home screen evident on the display. All you need to do now is open the app and get started.

In **Fig. 4.2**, you can see the opened app, and have the basic digital SLM display running, reading 51.2 dB. This was the sound level (dBA) with light background music playing. It's a nice, big display, but to share this information, a screen shot is needed. Fortunately, this is very easy to do, and once you've learned the trick, you'll use it for many other purposes. To get a screen shot on an iOS device, simply hold down the "Home" button on the front of the device while simultaneously pressing the "On/Off" button on the top. The screen will flash, and if you have the sound turned on, a camera shutter sound will be audible. You have now saved a screen shot of your measurement to the Camera Roll in the Photos file on your iOS device—perfect!

Below, in **Figs. 4.3** and **4.4**, you can see screen shots taken from an iPhone in the "Portrait" screen orientation. **Figure 4.3** shows an analog SLM representation, and **Fig. 4.4** shows a digital SLM. Of note in **Fig. 4.4** is that, from the "dashboard" of the app, one may

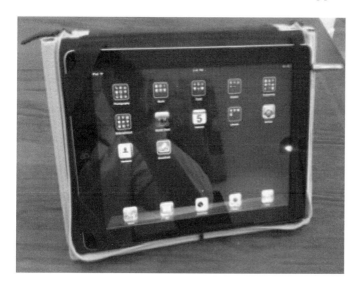

Fig. 4.1   iPad with MicW i436 connected (top right corner).

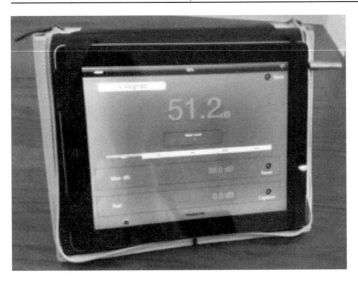

Fig. 4.2   iPad with Digital Sound Level Meter app running.

select various performance parameters of the SLM while the app is running, and on the top left corner you can see that "A Weighted" has been chosen as the weighting scheme. Most other weighting options are available, of course.

While SLM screen shots are clear and somewhat informative, a more powerful metric would be to conduct a sound study over time. Now we are getting to the really useful applications directly related to measuring the acoustical aspects of a classroom according to the ANSI S-12.6 2010 Standard. **Figure 4.5** shows a sound study conducted in an unoccupied classroom. Notice it is time stamped, and LEQ is also noted in the top, right corner. This is a much more illustrative graph to share with other stakeholders compared with a simple SLM screen shot, as it shows SPL over time and documentation of the date and time the measurement was taken, as well as the duration of the measurement. In this case, ~3 minutes, 30 seconds of data were collected, with ~1 minute, 18 seconds shown in the displayed screen shot. It is interesting to note that this particular classroom nearly meets the ANSI standard for unoccupied classrooms of 35 dBA. Yes, it can be done!

If we simply conduct several sound studies at various locations in the classroom and take screen shots in each location, we have a very powerful set of illustrations to share regarding the unoccupied noise levels of the enclosure.

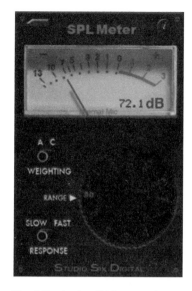
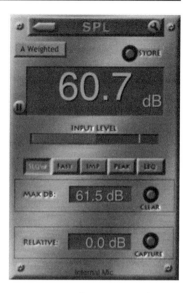

Fig. 4.3 Analog SLM screen shot.   **Fig. 4.4** Digital SLM screen shot.

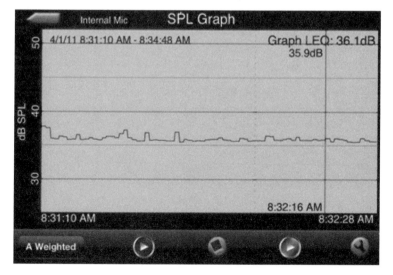

Fig. 4.5 Sound study graph of an unoccupied classroom.

What about reverberation measures? In the bundle of apps on AudioTools is an "Impulse Response" feature. This is where octave band RT60 measures are obtained. There are several ways to do this and Studio Six Digital has a good video tutorial on the subject. For best results, a swept sine wave should be used as a source. However, this requires audio playback equipment capable of producing a wide bandwidth signal at fairly high sound pressure levels and may not be practical in all cases. A simple impulse signal, for example a handclap or balloon pop, is generally all that is needed as a signal source to allow the Impulse Response feature to extrapolate accurate RT60 measures at the desired octave bands.

Figure 4.6 shows the Energy Time Curve (ETC) obtained in the same classroom in which the unoccupied sound study data shown in **Fig. 4.5** were collected. While it does display the energy decay over time within the enclosure, it does not provide the RT60 measures needed for comparison to the ANSI standard.

Simply clicking on the "ETC" icon causes a popup menu to appear that allows us to select RT60 measurements (labeled in this earlier version AudioTools as "T30"). **Figure 4.7** shows the octave band RT60 measurements for this classroom. Of note is that this is a fairly

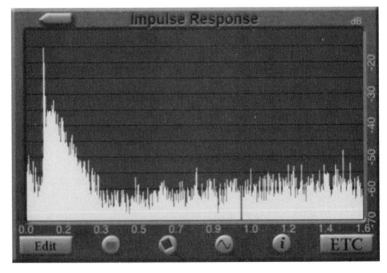

Fig. 4.6 Energy time curve of an unoccupied classroom.

non-reverberant enclosure. Indeed it does meet the ANSI standard. (The absence of measures in octave bands at lower frequencies is related to the intensity of the impulse. A balloon pop may have yielded data at lower frequencies compared with a handclap.) The decrease in reverberation time as frequency increases is expected.

We now have obtained the core data needed to compare the acoustical characteristics of a given classroom with the ANSI standard. We have succeeded in doing so accurately, quickly, affordably, and in a manner that allows us to share the information in an email to other stakeholders. Simply drag and drop the screen shots into the body of the email, and the data are sent in full color to the desired recipients along with the necessary narrative explanation.

The entire process of measuring the basic acoustical properties of a classroom in accordance with ANSI recommendations, as well as formatting/sending an email with a supplemental report that includes clear graphical representation of the data, can be completed in less than 30 minutes, and conducted entirely from your smart phone or other hand-held device. Wow! There may even be time remaining to shop for a nice, ripe watermelon!

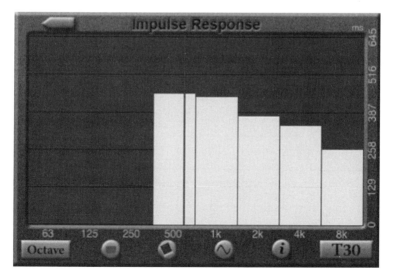

Fig. 4.7 RT60 measures displayed in octave bands.

◆ Appendix 4.1
Classroom Acoustical Survey Worksheet[1]

Date _____ Audiologist/Surveyor _____

School Room Teacher _____

Student Name (if applicable) _____ Grade _____

This worksheet is intended to be used to screen for acoustical problems in classrooms. When noise and/or reverberation levels are suspected to exceed those recommended by ANSI/ASA S12.60 (2009/2010), the screening survey data are an indicator for further assessment. This assessment may include a referral to an acoustical specialist who can perform a comprehensive acoustical analysis and suggest solutions.

SECTION 1: Background Noise Measurements

Classroom Schematic Diagram: <u>see attached</u>

Sound Level Meter: Make/Model# _____

Method Used: ☐ One Hour Average
　　　　　　　☐ Short-Term: ____ second average; # of time samples ____

Background Noise Levels (dBA, dBC)
Unoccupied & Occupied Classroom

circle number for condition:		1=unoccupied, HVAC off 3=occupied, HVAC off		2=unoccupied, HVAC on 4=occupied, HVAC on			
		1　2　3　4		1　2　3　4		1　2　3　4	1　2　3　4
Decibel Weighting		dBA	dBC	dBA	dBC	dBA	dBC	dBA	dBC
Measurement Locations	**L1***								
	L2								
	L3								
	L4								
	L5								
	L6								
Average dB Level:									

*Target Student

---

[1]*Source:* Adapted from J. J. Smaldino, C. C. Crandell, & B. M. Kreisman (2005). Acoustic measurements in classrooms. In C. C. Crandell, J. J. Smaldino, & C. Flexer (Eds.), *Sound field amplification: Applications to speech perception and classroom acoustics* (2nd ed., p. 131). Clifton Park, NY: Delmar Cengage Learning.

SECTION 2: Reverberation Time (RT60)

Measured RT60: _____ Sound stimulus used: _____

Measuring instrumentation used: _____

Frequency:		500 Hz	1000 Hz	2000 Hz
Measurement Locations	RT1			
	RT2			
	RT3			
	RT4			
	Middle			
RT60 Ave Second per frequency:				

Overall RT-60 Classroom Average
(RT60 at 500, 1000, 2000 Hz) : _____ seconds

Estimated RT60:

Note: On-line RT60 calculation programs may also be used for this calculation
(e.g., www.sengpielaudio.com/calculator-RT60.htm, www.mcsquared.com/
homerteng.htm).

Room Volume (V) = cubic feet

Area Floor × ABS. Coef. = A Floor

Area Ceiling × ABS. Coef. = A Ceiling

Area Side Wall 1 × ABS. Coef. = A Wall 1

Area Side Wall 2 × ABS. Coef. = A Wall 2

Area End Wall 1 × ABS. Coef. = A End 1

Area End Wall 2 × ABS. Coef. = A End 2

Total A

Estimated Average Classroom RT60 = $0.049 \times (V) / (A)$ = _____ seconds

SECTION 3: Estimate of Critical Distance

Using **Table 4.2** provided in the chapter, match the volume and estimated
reverberation time of the room being analyzed. The resulting value is the critical distance.

The authors wish to thank Andrew Smith of Studio Six Digital for technical information about Apple iPhone/iPad performance parameters.

References

American National Standards Institute (ANSI/ASA) (2009/2010). ANSI/ASA S12.60-2010 American National Standard Acoustical Performance Criteria, Design Requirements, and Guidelines for Schools, Part 1: Permanent Schools, and Part 2: Relocatable Classrooms Factors. New York: American National Standards Institute. Available at http://asastore.aip.org

ANSI/ASA (2002). ANSI/ASA S12.60-2002 American National Standard Acoustical Performance Criteria, Design Requirements, and Guidelines for Schools. New York: American National Standards Institute.

Berg, F. S. (1993). *Acoustics and sound systems in the schools.* San Diego, CA: Singular Publishing Group.

Bess, F. H., Sinclair, J. S., & Riggs, D. E. (1984, May-June). Group amplification in schools for the hearing impaired. *Ear and Hearing, 5*(3), 138–144.

Crandell, C. C., & Smaldino, J. J. (1995). An update of classroom acoustics for children with hearing impairment. *The Volta Review, 6,* 18–25.

Sanders, D. A. (1965, March). Noise conditions in normal school classrooms. *Exceptional Children, 31,* 344–353.

Sato, H., & Bradley, J. S. (2008, April). Evaluation of acoustical conditions for speech communication in working elementary school classrooms. *The Journal of the Acoustical Society of America, 123*(4), 2064–2077.

5 Classroom Audio Distribution Systems: Literature Review 2003–2011

Andrew B. John and Brian M. Kreisman

Scientific reports on the efficacy of the classroom audio distribution system (CADS) have been available to audiologists and educators since the mid-1980s. The period since 2000 has seen a rapid increase in the rate of publication for these studies, providing interested parties with a wealth of evidence to support the use of these technologies in the classroom. Among the best resources on this topic is the excellent review conducted by Gail Gegg Rosenberg (2005) covering the literature on this tool from its inception to 2003. The present review is intended to supplement that resource by evaluating research pertinent to CADS published primarily in the period from 2003 to 2011. See Appendix 5.1 for a table that summarizes all reviewed articles. In addition, the reader is directed to Rosenberg's (2005) chapter for information on earlier studies, including the foundational work that led to the research cited here.

◆ Research on Classroom Acoustic Environments

Recent studies have affirmed decades of research attesting to the detrimental acoustic environments found in typical classrooms. In two such evaluations, Pugh, Miura, and Asahara (2006) and Nelson, Smaldino, Erler, and Garstecki (2008) measured background noise levels in unoccupied elementary school classrooms. Background noise levels in all classrooms examined in these two investigations were above the 35 dBA criterion recommended by the *American National Standard Acoustical Performance Criteria, Design Requirements, and Guidelines for Schools* (ANSI S12.60-2010). Choi and McPherson (2005) reported background noise levels in occupied mainstream primary classrooms in Hong Kong as averaging 61 dBA, while Massie and Dillon (2006a) reported occupied noise levels ranging from 64 to 72 dBA in Australian primary school classrooms. In addition to these data reported on mainstream classes, Leung and McPherson (2006) found mean unoccupied noise levels of 36 to 52 dBA in eight Hong Kong classrooms for children with developmental disabilities. Compounding the issue of high noise levels in the learning environment is the fact that cooperative learning activities, which may provide both educational and social benefits, tend to increase the noise level in the classroom (Whitlock & Dodd, 2008). Latham and Blumsack (2008) reported results from a survey of educational audiologists on acoustical features of classrooms. Common sources of ambient noise cited were heating, ventilation, and air conditioning (HVAC) systems; movable desks and chairs; overhead projectors; and classroom computers. Most audiologists reported that HVAC noise was likely to be loud enough to interfere with listening to the teacher. Reflective architectural features, including drywall and cinderblock walls, drapeless windows, and hard flooring, were also reported by many respondents.

◆ Speech Perception Studies

The effect of these poor acoustical environments is seen in measures of speech intelligibility by children listening in class. Jamieson, Kranjc, Yu, and Hodgetts (2004) and Bradley and Sato (2008) have reported significant effects of age (older children outperform younger children) and background noise (higher noise levels result in decreased intelligibility) on speech understanding. Bradley and Sato noted that, in their study, the youngest children showed significantly decreased speech intelligibility in the presence of noise even at a +15 dB signal-to-noise ratio (SNR), a level that would be considered very good in most classrooms (ANSI, 2010).

Reverberation in the presence of noise has also been shown to degrade speech perception in classrooms. Studies by Klatte, Lachmann, and Meis (2010) and Neuman, Wroblewski, Hajicek, and Rubinstein (2010) reported that elementary school–age children show speech perception declines in the presence of typical classroom levels of noise and reverberation, and that those declines are significantly greater than those seen in adults. Notably, the participants in Klatte's study self-reported that the noise and reverberation in the classroom did not prevent them from hearing and understanding speech. This finding suggests that the interference with understanding caused by a poor acoustic environment may be underrated by children in an informal evaluation of the classroom.

◆ Level of Effort

The effects of room acoustics on understanding can also be measured by assessing the effort required to listen and understand in that room. Howard, Munro, and Plack (2010) found that listening effort is significantly increased in children listening to speech in a background of children's chatter at typical SNRs found in classrooms (quiet, +4, 0, and –4 dB) while undertaking a secondary task (rehearsing digit sequences). A significant effect of SNR was found for the digit rehearsal task, suggesting that as noise in the classroom increases, children may lose the ability to multitask or perform effortful learning activities.

These data are consistent with those reported for previous decades and elsewhere in this handbook: the classroom environment is typically loud, reverberant, and poorly acoustically managed. It is therefore not surprising to find studies conducted after implementation of the ANSI 12.60-2010 classroom acoustic guidelines (initially published in 2002) that continue to report diminished speech perception in poor acoustic classroom environments.

◆ Research on Classroom Audio Distribution Systems (CADS)

There is ample evidence that the poor acoustics of many classrooms can be ameliorated using classroom amplification systems. In one study, installation of sound-field frequency-modulated (FM) amplification systems and public address (PA) systems resulted in SNRs of +24 and +20, respectively, in eight classrooms in Hong Kong (Leung & McPherson, 2006). The average output from both systems met the recommended level of +15 dB and represented a significant improvement over the SNRs measured in the same classrooms without CADS. Notably, the FM system provided a statistically significantly better SNR than the PA system and reached +15 dB SNR in all classrooms measured, compared with six of eight for the PA system. Massie and Dillon (2006a) reported that sound-field FM amplification resulted in SNRs ranging from +4 to +10 across several noisy (64–72 dBA occupied) classrooms in Australia.

Similar positive results have been demonstrated with infrared CADS technology: Larsen and Blair (2008) found that when school was in session, students in five classrooms could hear a teacher's voice at a +13 SNR when a sound-field infrared system was in use, compared with +2 when the system was turned off. A paper by Larsen, Vega, and Ribera (2008) reported that an infrared CADS improved perception of single-syllable words in two college classrooms, one that met ANSI S12.60 recommendations and one that did not. Intelligibility was significantly better in the ANSI-compliant classroom, but students in both rooms benefited from installation of the infrared system. Millett and Purcell (2010) evaluated the benefit of infrared CADS in 12 first-grade classrooms in Canada in comparison with 12 classrooms without CADS. This study identified a greater change in the percentage of students reading at grade level over one year in the CADS-equipped classrooms, as well as a trend toward improved reading outcomes for students at risk for reading difficulty, though changes were not statistically significant.

Educational Benefit of CADS

In addition to speech perception improvement, CADS has been shown to improve learning and social behaviors of children in classrooms where such systems are in use. Massie, Theodoros, McPherson, and Smaldino (2004) described several benefits of sound-field amplification in classes of Aboriginal and Torres Strait Islander children in Australia. These benefits included increases in communicative activity with peers and teachers, as well as an increased rate of unprompted spoken interactions overall. The authors note that this increased participation in the classroom is likely to lead to better educational outcomes.

Indeed, recent studies have identified associations between use of CADS and measured educational achievement. Studies have found that elementary school students in amplified classrooms demonstrated improvement in skills including literacy, reading fluency, listening comprehension, and reading vocabulary, resulting in improved standardized test scores compared with peers in unamplified classrooms (Chelius, 2004; Gertel, McCarty, & Schoff, 2004; Heeney, 2007). Heeney reported on a study of 30 classrooms in New Zealand in which sound-field amplification systems were installed. Results suggest that, with appropriate configuration of equipment, use of the amplification systems over the course of a year resulted in improved overall academic achievement by students, including better listening performance and improved scores on literacy tasks that assess reading comprehension and vocabulary. A study in Canada by Langlan, Sockalingam, Caissie, and Kreisman (2009) similarly found that use of classroom sound-field FM amplification led to increases in academic achievement, communication, class behavior, participation, and attention. Attention showed the greatest increase when sound-field amplification was employed, suggesting that improvements in this skill are particularly attainable with listening technology.

Regular use of CADS during daily classroom activities may also provide educators with better data for assessing educational progress. Studies by Taub, Kanis, and Kramer (2003) and by Pinard (2006) both describe improvements in scores obtained on the Screening Instrument for Targeting Educational Risk (SIFTER) after installation of sound-field amplification. Taub and colleagues, who evaluated children in a low-socioeconomic-status urban classroom environment, note that provision of appropriate amplification may lead to better identification of children at risk for academic difficulty.

The benefits provided by CADS have also been demonstrated for other populations, including children speaking English as a second language, children with attention deficit hyperactivity disorder (ADHD), and children in special education classes. Massie and Dillon (2006a) reported a benefit of sound-field amplification for listening and academic skill areas (including reading and writing) that was consistent for children who did and did not speak English as a first language. In contrast, Nelson, Kohnert, Sabur, and Shaw (2005) did not find an improvement in speech perception or on-task behavior among second-graders for whom English was the second language when a sound-field amplification system was in use. The authors suggest that appropriate acoustical treatment of the classrooms in which the study took place may have improved outcomes.

Maag and Anderson (2007) evaluated the effects of CADS on the speed at which three elementary school students with ADHD responded to teacher commands. Following introduction of the amplification system, improvements were seen for all tasks evaluated, including difficult tasks, such as understanding multiple instructions given simultaneously. Flexer and Long (2003) reported that special education referral rates in the Oconto Falls, Wisconsin, school district dropped from an average of 7.72 percent during 1989–1998 to 4.6 percent for 1998–2000, after installation of a sound-field amplification system in every K–5 classroom in the district. While more research is needed into the specific benefits of CADS in populations with learning disabilities or delays, these data suggest this technology as a low-cost improvement for both mainstream and special education classrooms that may substantially reduce costly over-referrals to specialized classes.

Teacher Benefits of CADS

A large number of studies have reported on teacher preference for CADS, including studies describing potential vocal health benefits for the teacher when an amplification system is used regularly. For example, a series of studies by Jónsdottir (2002) and colleagues (2001, 2002, 2003) describe the effect of portable amplification systems on vocal quality and strain among teachers in Iceland. These studies found that use of amplification systems decreased vocal load (Jónsdottir, Rantala, Laukkanen, & Vilkman, 2001) and led to improvements in self-reported ease of speaking and vocal endurance (Jónsdottir, 2002) as well as decreased fatigue (Jónsdottir, Laukkanen, & Siikki, 2003). Evaluations conducted objectively by analysis of teachers' fundamental frequency and sound pressure levels produced across the day (Jónsdottir, Laukkanen, & Vilkman, 2002) and subjectively by speech trainer ratings (Jónsdottir et al., 2003) confirmed improvement in vocal quality and decreased vocal load.

Other studies have produced similar results: Edwards and Fuen (2005) found that school teachers using CADS reported less vocal strain and greater voice clarity compared with experiences without amplification. Massie and Dillon (2006b) also found that teachers reported reduced vocal strain when a sound-field amplification system was in use, and that teachers' voices were perceived as better, clearer, or louder by students when the system was in use. Morrow and Connor (2011) used ambulatory phonation monitoring and analysis to assess elementary school music teachers' vocal load. Analysis revealed significant decreases in vocal intensity and phonation time when amplification was in use, which reduced overall vocal load. These results support previous findings of significantly decreased strain on teachers' voices when CADS is in use.

Other benefits of CADS aside from vocal health benefit are reported by classroom teachers as well. Students in Icelandic classrooms reported that listening and concentration were easier when the teacher used an amplification system (Jónsdottir, 2002). A survey of Australian teachers by Massie and Dillon (2006b) found that teachers observed improvement in students' attention, communication, and classroom behavior when amplification systems were in use. Rubin, Aquino-Rusell, and Flagg-Williams (2007) conducted a study of 60 Canadian classrooms, grades 1–3, approximately half of which were equipped with sound-field amplification systems. Compared with students in classrooms without amplification, students in amplified classrooms showed significant increases in responses to teacher statements, decreases in requests for the teacher to repeat commands and questions, and decreases in student cross-talk when the teacher was giving instructions. As a result, teachers needed to use less time to direct and maintain students' attention and reported that students were more engaged in learning. Similarly, Ryan (2009) found that use of a portable sound-field amplification system led to increased productivity for two middle school physical education teachers as a result of a reduction in time needed for organizational and transitional class activities.

Negative or Non-Significant Findings

Mention of some negative results in recent studies of CADS is warranted. Anderson and Goldstein (2004) evaluated eight children ages 9–12 with mild to severe hearing loss using personal FM systems coupled to hearing aids, desktop personal FM systems, and an infrared sound-field system. Benefit was seen with use of the two personal FM systems but not the infrared sound-field system. In a follow-up study, Anderson, Goldstein, Colodzin, and Iglehart (2005) compared personal, desk-mounted, and sound-field FM systems used by 28 children ages 8–14 with hearing aids or a cochlear implant. While speech intelligibility improvements were seen across all amplification systems compared with listening with hearing aids or implant alone, significantly better performance was seen using desk-level and personal FM systems coupled with children's own amplification devices. In addition, a large majority (26 of 28) of the participants expressed a preference for the desk or personal FM system over the sound-field system.

Other studies have noted a lack of CADS benefit for users of cochlear implants (CI). A meta-analysis by Schafer and Kleinek (2009) found that sound-field amplification systems provided no significant speech recognition benefit over CI use alone. Benefit was seen for direct-audio-input (DAI) FM systems coupled with CI, leading the authors to suggest that audiologists should recommend directly coupled amplification systems for classroom use by children with such implants. Another study by Iglehart (2004) did find improved speech perception by children using CI with desktop and sound-field FM systems, but no difference between the two types in a quiet room, and an advantage for the desktop system in noisy rooms. More research is needed in this area, but existing data may not support CADS benefits for children who use CI.

Sound-field amplification is not appropriate for all classroom acoustic environments. Wilson, Marinac, Pitty, and Burrows (2011) reported that infrared CADS installation in a permanent classroom resulted in small but significant improvements in listening and auditory analysis for children ages 7 to 9 in some, but not all, Australian classrooms examined. Classrooms in schools with lower background noise and reverberation times tended to show more benefit from the amplification system, leading the authors to suggest that sound-field amplification may not be beneficial in acoustically unsuitable rooms such as an open classroom plan. For a discussion of appropriate noise control and strategies to maximize intelligibility in open-plan classroom environments, see Shield, Greenland, and Dockrell (2010). Finally, Lubman (2008) argues that provision of classroom amplification should never be regarded as a substitute for appropriate noise control in classrooms.

Additional Research Needed

Additional research is needed in several areas pertaining to classroom acoustics and amplification, including longitudinal studies of CADS efficacy and comparisons among various sound-field technologies currently available to educators. In addition, more study is needed on the potential benefit of CADS in special populations such as children with auditory processing disorder, language delay, and learning disabilities. Several real-life variables also complicate the study of CADS benefit and limit the ecological validity of research findings with these systems. Presently there is limited research evaluating factors such as teacher training (including expert in-service), microphone use, the role of pass-around microphones, and the potential interaction of personal FM and CADS used in the same space. Future studies may provide better understanding of the factors that may limit success with CADS and provide strategies for educational audiologists to ensure the positive outcomes seen in the studies cited here and reported anecdotally every day.

Appendix 5.1 Summary of Recent Research on CADS and Related Topics, 2003–2011

Author	Year	Title	Summary of Selected Findings
American National Standards Institute (ANSI)	2010	American National Standard acoustical performance criteria, design requirements, and guidelines for schools	The standard describes recommendations for improving the listening environment in school classrooms.
Anderson and Goldstein	2004	Speech perception benefits of FM and infrared devices to children with hearing aids in a typical classroom	Children with hearing loss showed better speech perception using personal or desktop amplification systems than with CADS.
Anderson et al.	2005	Benefit of S/N enhancing devices to speech perception of children listening in a typical classroom with hearing aids or a cochlear implant	Children with hearing aids or cochlear implants demonstrated better speech intelligibility using coupled personal or desktop amplification systems than with CADS.
Bradley and Sato	2008	The intelligibility of speech in elementary school classrooms	Higher noise levels decreased school-age children's understanding of speech in the classroom, particularly for the youngest children.
Chelius	2004	Trost amplification study	Use of CADS resulted in improved educational achievement outcomes.
Choi and McPherson	2005	Noise levels in Hong Kong primary schools: Implications for classroom listening	High levels of noise were measured in mainstream primary school classrooms in Hong Kong.
Edwards and Fuen	2005	A formative evaluation of sound-field amplification system across several grade levels in four schools	Teachers using CADS reported decreased vocal strain and greater voice clarity.
Flexer and Long	2003	Sound-field amplification: Preliminary information regarding special education referrals	Special education referral rates in a Wisconsin school district decreased after installation of CADS in all K–5 classrooms.

Author	Year	Title	Summary of Selected Findings
Gertel et al.	2004	High performance schools equals high performing students	Use of CADS increased standardized test scores in elementary school classrooms.
Heeney	2007	Classroom sound field amplification, listening, and learning	Appropriately configured CADS improved academic achievement and literacy in 30 New Zealand classrooms.
Howard et al.	2010	Listening effort at signal-to-noise ratios that are typical of the school classroom	Increased background noise caused greater effort to be expended during listening and limited the ability of children to multi-task.
Iglehart	2004	Speech perception by students with cochlear implants using sound-field systems in classrooms	Both CADS and desktop amplification systems increased speech perception by children with cochlear implants, but desktop systems showed the greatest advantage.
Jamieson et al.	2004	Speech intelligibility of young school-aged children in the presence of real-life classroom noise	Higher noise levels decreased school-age children's understanding of speech in the classroom.
Jónsdottir	2002	Cordless amplifying system in classrooms	Use of CADS led to improvement in ease of speaking and vocal endurance among teachers; students reported easier listening and concentration with CADS in use.
Jónsdottir et al.	2001	Effects of sound amplification on teachers' speech while teaching	Use of CADS may decrease teacher vocal load.

Author	Year	Title	Summary of Selected Findings
Jónsdottir et al.	2002	Changes in teachers' speech during a working day with and without electric sound amplification	Measurement of teacher voice characteristics using CADS throughout the day showed improved vocal quality and decreased vocal load.
Jónsdottir et al.	2003	Changes in teachers' voice quality during a working day with and without electric sound amplification	Teachers reported decreased fatigue when using CADS.
Klatte et al.	2010	Effects of noise and reverberation on speech perception and listening comprehension of children and adults in a classroom-like setting	Speech perception declines were seen in the presence of increased noise and reverberation in the classroom.
Langlan et al.	2009	The benefit of sound-field amplification in First Nations elementary school children in Nova Scotia, Canada	Use of CADS resulted in increased academic achievement and improvements in communication and attention in a First Nations elementary school in Canada.
Larsen and Blair	2008	The effect of classroom amplification on the signal-to-noise ratio in classrooms while class is in session	CADS significantly improved SNR in five classrooms.
Larsen et al.	2008	The effect of room acoustics and sound-field amplification on word recognition performance in young adult listeners in suboptimal listening conditions	CADS significantly improved speech perception in ANSI-compliant and non–ANSI-compliant college classrooms.
Latham and Blumsack	2008	Classroom acoustics: A survey of educational audiologists	Several classroom factors contributing to high levels of noise and reverberation are identified by educational audiologists.

Author	Year	Title	Summary of Selected Findings
Leung and McPherson	2006	Classrooms for children with developmental disabilities: Sound-field and public address amplification systems compared	High levels of noise were measured in classrooms for children with developmental disabilities in Hong Kong; significant improvements in SNR were seen after installation of CADS.
Lubman	2008	Sound field amplification competes with noise control	Appropriate noise control and acoustical modification of the classroom should precede installation of any CADS.
Maag and Anderson	2007	Sound-field amplification to increase compliance to directions in students with ADHD	Three children with ADHD showed improved response to teacher commands with CADS in use.
Massie and Dillon	2006a	The impact of sound-field amplification in mainstream cross-cultural classrooms, Part 1: Educational outcomes	High levels of noise were measured in primary school classrooms in Australia; improvements were seen following installation of CADS.
Massie and Dillon	2006b	The impact of sound-field amplification in mainstream cross-cultural classrooms, Part 2: Teacher and child opinions	Teachers using CADS reported decreased vocal strain; students confirmed greater clarity and loudness and showed improved behavior with CADS in use.
Massie et al.	2004	Sound-field amplification: Enhancing the classroom listening environment for Aboriginal and Torres Strait Islander children	Use of CADS significantly increased communicative behaviors in Aboriginal and Torres Strait Islander classrooms in Australia.
Millet and Purcell	2010	Effect of sound field amplification on grade 1 reading outcomes	Trends toward improved reading outcomes were seen following installation of CADS in Canadian first-grade classrooms.

Author	Year	Title	Summary of Selected Findings
Morrow and Connor	2011	Voice amplification as a means of reducing vocal load for elementary music teachers	Using CADS decreased teachers' vocal load and phonation time.
Nelson, E. L., et al.	2008	Background noise levels and reverberation times in old and new elementary school classrooms	Classroom noise and reverberation levels exceeded ANSI recommendations.
Nelson, P., et al.	2005	Classroom noise and children learning through a second language: Double jeopardy?	CADS did not significantly improve speech perception or on-task behavior in a classroom of students for whom English was a second language.
Neuman et al.	2010	Combined effects of noise and reverberation on speech recognition performance of normal-hearing children and adults	Speech perception declines were seen in the presence of increased noise and reverberation in the classroom.
Pinard	2006	Prevalence of otitis media and hearing loss and effects of sound-field FM amplification among First Nations elementary school children	Improvements on the SIFTER were seen following use of CADS in a First Nations elementary school in Canada.
Pugh et al.	2006	Noise levels among first, second, and third grade elementary school classrooms in Hawai'i	Classroom noise levels exceeded ANSI recommendations.
Rosenberg	2005	Sound field amplification: A comprehensive literature review	Research findings in studies of classroom acoustics and CADS prior to 2004 are reviewed.
Rubin et al.	2007	Evaluating sound field amplification technology in New Brunswick schools	Use of CADS in Canadian elementary classrooms resulted in significant increases in student responses to questions and decreases in requests for repetition and student cross-talk.

Author	Year	Title	Summary of Selected Findings
Ryan	2009	The effects of a sound-field amplification system on managerial time in middle school physical education settings	Use of portable CADS reduced managerial time in two physical education classrooms.
Schafer and Kleineck	2009	Improvements in speech-recognition performance using cochlear implants and three types of FM systems: A meta-analytic approach	Children with cochlear implants using directly coupled amplification showed greater speech intelligibility improvements than with CADS.
Shield et al.	2010	Noise in open plan classrooms in primary schools: A review	Appropriate acoustical modification for open-plan classrooms is discussed.
Taub et al.	2003	Reducing acoustic barriers in classrooms: A report comparing two kindergarten classrooms in an inner-city school	Regular use of CADS resulted in significant improvements on the SIFTER in a low-socioeconomic-status urban classroom.
Whitlock and Dodd	2008	Speech intelligibility in classrooms: Specific acoustical needs for primary school children	Cooperative learning activities tend to increase the ambient noise level in classrooms, creating a poorer environment for understanding speech.
Wilson et al.	2011	The use of sound-field amplification devices in different types of classrooms	Children showed small but significant improvements in listening and auditory skills using CADS, but some classrooms were unsuitable for the technology.

References

American National Standards Institute (ANSI). (2010). *American National Standard acoustical performance criteria, design requirements, and guidelines for schools, Parts 1 and 2* (ANSI S12.60-2010). New York, NY: Acoustical Society of America.

Anderson, K. L., & Goldstein, H. (2004, April). Speech perception benefits of FM and infrared devices to children with hearing aids in a typical classroom. *Language, Speech, and Hearing Services in Schools, 35*(2), 169–184.

Anderson, K., Goldstein, H., Colodzin, L., & Iglehart, F. (2005). Benefit of S/N enhancing devices to speech perception of children listening in a typical classroom with hearing aids or a cochlear implant. *Journal of Educational Audiology, 12,* 14–28.

Bradley, J. S., & Sato, H. (2008, April). The intelligibility of speech in elementary school classrooms. *Journal of the Acoustical Society of America, 123*(4), 2078–2086.

Chelius, L. (2004). Trost amplification study (unpublished report, Canby, OR, School District).

Choi, Y. C., & McPherson, B. (2005). Noise levels in Hong Kong primary schools: Implications for classroom listening. *International Journal of Disability Development and Education, 52*(4), 345–360.

Edwards, D., & Fuen, L. (2005). A formative evaluation of sound-field amplification system across several grade levels in four schools. *Journal of Educational Audiology, 12,* 59–66.

Flexer, C., & Long, S. (2003). Sound-field amplification: Preliminary information regarding special education referrals. *Communication Disorders Quarterly, 25,* 29–34.

Gertel, S., McCarty, P., & Schoff, L. (2004). High performance schools equals high performing students. *Educational Facility Planner, 39*(3), 20–24.

Heeney, M. (2007). Classroom sound field amplification, listening, and learning (unpublished dissertation, University of Newcastle, NSW, Australia).

Howard, C. S., Munro, K. J., & Plack, C. J. (2010, December). Listening effort at signal-to-noise ratios that are typical of the school classroom. *International Journal of Audiology, 49*(12), 928–932.

Iglehart, F. (2004, June). Speech perception by students with cochlear implants using sound-field systems in classrooms. *American Journal of Audiology, 13*(1), 62–72.

Jamieson, D. G., Kranjc, G., Yu, K., & Hodgetts, W. E. (2004, July–August). Speech intelligibility of young school-aged children in the presence of real-life classroom noise. *Journal of the American Academy of Audiology, 15*(7), 508–517.

Jónsdottir, V. I. (2002). Cordless amplifying system in classrooms: A descriptive study of teachers' and students' opinions. *Logopedics, Phoniatrics, Vocology, 27*(1), 29–36.

Jónsdottir, V., Laukkanen, A. M., & Siikki, I. (2003, September–October). Changes in teachers' voice quality during a working day with and without electric sound amplification. *Folia Phoniatrica et Logopaedica, 55*(5), 267–280.

Jónsdottir, V., Laukkanen, A. M., & Vilkman, E. (2002, November–December). Changes in teachers' speech during a working day with and without electric sound amplification. *Folia Phoniatrica et Logopaedica, 54*(6), 282–287.

Jónsdottir, V., Rantala, L., Laukkanen, A. M., & Vilkman, E. (2001). Effects of sound amplification on teachers' speech while teaching. *Logopedics, Phoniatrics, Vocology, 26*(3), 118–123.

Klatte, M., Lachmann, T., & Meis, M. (2010, October–December). Effects of noise and reverberation on speech perception and listening comprehension of children and adults in a classroom-like setting. *Noise and Health: Special Issue on Noise: Memory and Learning, 12*(49), 270–282.

Langlan, L., Sockalingam, R., Caissie, R., & Kreisman, B. M. (2009). The benefit of sound-field amplification in First Nations elementary school children in Nova Scotia, Canada. *Australian and New Zealand Journal of Audiology, 31,* 55–71.

Larsen, J. B., & Blair, J. C. (2008, October). The effect of classroom amplification on the signal-to-noise ratio in classrooms while class is in session. *Language, Speech, and Hearing Services in Schools, 39*(4), 451–460.

Larsen, J. B., Vega, A., & Ribera, J. E. (2008, June). The effect of room acoustics and sound-field amplification on word recognition performance in young adult listeners in suboptimal listening conditions. *American Journal of Audiology, 17*(1), 50–59.

Latham, N. M., & Blumsack, J. T. (2008). Classroom acoustics: A survey of educational audiologists. *Journal of Educational Audiology, 14,* 58–69.

Leung, S. W. H., & McPherson, B. (2006). Classrooms for children with developmental disabilities: Sound-field and public address amplification systems compared. *International Journal of Disability Development and Education, 53*(3), 287–299.

Lubman, D. (2008). *Sound field amplification competes with noise control.* Paper presented at the 156th meeting of the Acoustical Society of America, Miami, FL.

Maag, J. W., & Anderson, J. M. (2007). Sound-field amplification to increase compliance to directions in students with ADHD. *Behavioral Disorders, 32*(4), 238–253.

Massie, R., & Dillon, H. (2006a). The impact of sound-field amplification in mainstream cross-cultural classrooms, Part 1: Educational outcomes. *Australian Journal of Education, 50*(1), 62–77.

Massie, R., & Dillon, H. (2006b). The impact of sound-field amplification in mainstream cross-cultural classrooms, Part 2: Teacher and child opinions. *Australian Journal of Education, 50*(1), 78–94.

Massie, R., Theodoros, D., McPherson, B., & Smaldino, J. J. (2004). Sound-field amplification: Enhancing the classroom listening environment for Aboriginal and Torres Strait Islander children. *Australian Journal of Indigenous Education, 33,* 47–53.

Millett, P., & Purcell, N. (2010). Effect of sound field amplification on grade 1 reading outcomes. *Canadian Journal of Speech-Language-Pathology and Audiology, 31*(4), 17–24.

Morrow, S. L., & Connor, N. P. (2011, July). Voice amplification as a means of reducing vocal load for elementary music teachers. *Journal of Voice, 25*(4), 441–446.

Nelson, E. L., Smaldino, J. J., Erler, S., & Garstecki, D. (2008). Background noise levels and reverberation times in old and new elementary school classrooms. *Journal of Educational Audiology, 14,* 16–22.

Nelson, P., Kohnert, K., Sabur, S., & Shaw, D. (2005, July). Classroom noise and children learning through a second language: Double jeopardy? *Language, Speech, and Hearing Services in Schools, 36*(3), 219–229.

Neuman, A. C., Wroblewski, M., Hajicek, J., & Rubinstein, A. (2010, June). Combined effects of noise and reverberation on speech recognition performance of normal-hearing children and adults. *Ear and Hearing, 31*(3), 336–344.

Pinard, L. (2006). Prevalence of otitis media and hearing loss and effects of sound-field FM amplification among First Nations elementary school children (unpublished master's thesis, Dalhousie University, Halifax, NS, Canada).

Pugh, K. C., Miura, C. A., & Asahara, L. L. Y. (2006). Noise levels among first, second, and third grade elementary school classrooms in Hawai'i. *Journal of Educational Audiology, 13,* 32–38.

Rosenberg, G. G. (2005). Sound field amplification: A comprehensive literature review. In C. C. Crandell, J. J. Smaldino, & C. Flexer (Eds.), *Sound field amplification: Applications to speech perception and classroom acoustics* (2nd Ed., pp. 72–111). Clifton Park, NY: Delmar Cengage Learning.

Rubin, R. L., Aquino-Rusell, C. E., & Flagg-Williams, J. (2007). *Evaluating sound field amplification technology in New Brunswick schools.* Paper presented at the 2007 conference of the Canadian Association of Speech-Language Pathologists and Audiologists.

Ryan, S. (2009, April). The effects of a sound-field amplification system on managerial time in middle school physical education settings. *Language, Speech, and Hearing Services in Schools, 40*(2), 131–137.

Schafer, E., & Kleinek, M. (2009). Improvements in speech-recognition performance using cochlear implants and three types of FM systems: A meta-analytic approach. *Journal of Educational Audiology, 15,* 4–14.

Shield, B., Greenland, E., & Dockrell, J. (2010, October–December). Noise in open plan classrooms in primary schools: A review. *Noise & Health, 12*(49), 225–234.

Taub, C. F., Kanis, R., & Kramer, L. (2003). Reducing acoustic barriers in classrooms: A report comparing two kindergarten classrooms in an inner-city school. *Journal of Educational Audiology, 11,* 69–74.

Whitlock, J. A. T., & Dodd, G. (2008). Speech intelligibility in classrooms: Specific acoustical needs for primary school children. *Building Acoustics, 15*(1), 35–47.

Wilson, W. J., Marinac, J., Pitty, K., & Burrows, C. (2011, October). The use of sound-field amplification devices in different types of classrooms. *Language, Speech, and Hearing Services in Schools, 42*(4), 395–407.

6 An Overview of Current CADS Technologies

Andrew B. John, Brian M. Kreisman, and Joseph J. Smaldino

◆ Introduction

The term "sound-field amplification system" has been traditionally used to refer to the small public address systems used to improve the signal-to-noise ratio (SNR) in the classroom. This term has been replaced with "classroom audio distribution system" (CADS). "Audio distribution system" is the common term for public address systems, so CADS is now the preferred way to refer to these systems in the classroom.

Once the audiologist or school administrator has determined the necessity for CADS in a classroom or school, the next step may be to select from the many CADS options presently available. This chapter is intended to provide an overview of current technology in CADS, including options for transmitters, receivers, and loudspeakers. Potential advantages and disadvantages of the major choices available will be detailed, and summary tables for each CADS technology are provided at the end of the chapter. It is our hope that this information will allow audiologists and educators to make informed decisions when selecting CADS for existing or new classrooms. The following descriptions are not exhaustive, but we hope that they will provide a starting point for individuals selecting a particular CADS.

The desired outcome with any CADS is an improvement in SNR (often of 8 dB or more) and an even distribution throughout the room of sound intensity and acoustic features that are important for speech perception. Options to accomplish this goal vary from compact, portable, battery-powered single-speaker units to more permanently placed, AC-powered speaker systems that use multiple traditional cone loudspeakers or employ some of the latest advances in speaker technology (Smaldino, 2011).

Generally speaking, CADS involves the use of a broadcasting microphone that the teacher and/or students use to transmit their voices to a compatible receiver and amplifier. The amplifier filters the received signal and carries it to one or more loudspeakers placed strategically in the classroom. **Figure 6.1** shows the components of a typical CADS.

Microphones typically include pendant, lapel, or head-worn boom microphones connected to a transmitting pack worn by the teacher. In some cases, hand-held "pass-around" microphones may be included to amplify students' voices while they ask or answer questions or during group discussions. Microphone types may include volume controls to modify the output level or may be adjusted automatically through circuitry in the transmitting unit. Most types of CADS employ a base receiver/amplifier device that receives the transmitted signal and routes it to a loudspeaker array. The receiver/amplifier may include volume controls as well as frequency-shaping options (such as a graphic equalizer) and connections for media devices and computers.

It is important to note that, prior to placement of any CADS, the classroom should be acoustically optimized using the techniques discussed in Chapter 4 of this handbook and elsewhere. Installation of CADS is not a substitute for acoustical treatment of the room. In fact, some studies have shown that CADS installed in acoustically inappropriate classrooms may provide little benefit or none at all (Iglehart, 2004; Wilson, Marinac, Pitty, & Burrows, 2011). Furthermore, we do not recommend any single CADS option as a solution

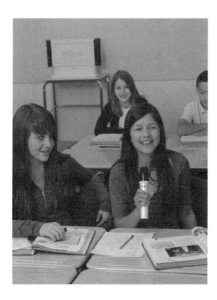

Fig. 6.1 Illustration of CADS.

for all classrooms. The choice of CADS should be a pragmatic one, taking into account room factors such as the size and shape of the room, the ambient noise and reverberation time of the room when in use, the number of students in the classroom, the need to interface with other technologies such as media players, as well as other room- or school-specific considerations.

Any CADS installation should be conducted carefully and thoughtfully and with appropriate follow-up by a consulting audiologist. In-service training of teachers and administrators is critical to the success of any CADS, regardless of the level of technology. At minimum, the daily maintenance of the system, instructions for charging batteries, and identification of whom to contact for repair or replacement of the system should be discussed and reinforced with all educators who will use the CADS.

There is an ample evidence base for the benefit of classroom amplification in terms of speech recognition, listening, attention, academic performance, and on-task behaviors (Lewis, 1991; Rosenberg, 2005; see also Chapter 5 of this handbook). In addition to these well-recognized benefits, CADS offers the added advantage of providing this amplification to all students in the classroom. This means that children with hearing loss, children with normal hearing, and children with other learning difficulties who may benefit from a better classroom SNR receive the advantages CADS can provide. Thus, the installation of CADS does not single out an individual child or group of children.

Teachers have reported several benefits of CADS use as well, including reductions in vocal strain and need for sick leave; less time needed for planning and transition time; and better attentiveness and behavior among students (Edwards & Fuen, 2005; Ryan, 2009; Sapienza, Crandell, & Curtis, 1999). Advances in classroom technology and use of digital media as a teaching tool provide yet another argument for a classroom amplification system that can interface with other systems to deliver academic content to students.

The choice of the most appropriate CADS for a single classroom, school, or school system should take into account several factors. These factors include the number of classrooms to be amplified, number of students per classroom, acoustical characteristics of each classroom, number and position of loudspeakers needed, number of microphones needed, flexibility and portability desired, need for in-service and follow-up maintenance, and use of other amplification devices (such as hearing aids and cochlear implants) by students. The next sections will address these and other considerations in the selection of CADS technology.

◆ Frequency Modulation (FM) Technology

Many existing CADS operate using wireless FM transmission. With an FM CADS, the acoustic voice signal of a talker is converted by the FM microphone to an electrical signal. That signal is transmitted wirelessly via a carrier wave modulated in the frequency domain. A receiver or multiple receivers tuned to the carrier frequency separate the signal from the carrier, amplify it, and present it to the room via one or more strategically placed loudspeakers.

Classroom FM systems have been used successfully in thousands of schools to enhance the SNR for students. A large research base has demonstrated the benefit of this technology for populations of children with hearing loss and those with normal hearing (Rosenberg, 2005; see also Chapter 5 of this handbook). In addition, large-scale studies have found FM CADS to be a cost-effective and efficient solution for the deleterious acoustical environment found in many classrooms (Rosenberg et al., 1999; Sarff, 1981).

There are several advantages to FM CADS. First, since these systems have been in wide use for many years, there are a large variety of manufacturers and systems from which to choose. This provides the educator or audiologist with significant flexibility with regard to number of microphones and loudspeakers, installation options, level of technological sophistication, and cost. Second, because line of sight is not necessary for FM transmission, signals do not drop out if either the transmitter or receiver moves in the classroom. Finally, FM CADS is a relatively inexpensive way to improve classroom speech perception. Typically priced less than similarly configured infrared CADS, FM CADS is a popular choice among school administrators who wish to provide an improved SNR to large classrooms without the cost of purchasing and maintaining a large number of personal FM devices.

Some potential disadvantages of FM CADS relate to the possibility of improper selection or installation. As noted above, it is critical to undertake an acoustical evaluation of the room to be amplified prior to installation of any CADS. An excessively noisy or reverberant room may limit or even eliminate the SNR benefit provided by an FM CADS variety. Second, an inappropriate number or arrangement of loudspeakers may limit the effectiveness of FM CADS. Speakers should be selected and positioned to provide as uniform a signal throughout the classroom as possible so that all children can take maximum advantage of the amplification provided.

Third, the narrow range of available frequencies for FM transmission and their relatively large transmission range limit effectiveness if this technology is used in multiple classrooms. These systems operate in the 216–217 MHz band. These frequencies have been assigned by the FCC for use with equipment by individuals with hearing loss. There is a finite number of narrow-band channels (typically about 20) in this frequency range. In order for the transmitter and receiver to operate as a system, they must be on the same frequency or channel. That is, each classroom must have its own frequencies assigned to it to prevent pickup of transmissions "spilling over" from nearby classrooms. At least two narrow-band frequencies are needed, for the teacher microphone and a separate "pass-around" microphone used by the students. It is easy to see that there would be enough frequencies to allow only a few FM CADS to be operating in proximity. Since the current trend is to improve the classroom SNR for all children, it is not uncommon for CADS to be needed in all of the classrooms within a school. Traditional FM-based systems are not ideal in this situation because of the limited frequency options. The exception is digital FM transmission, which will be discussed separately.

Finally, like many other CADS options, FM systems typically are not portable, limiting their benefit for students who use multiple classrooms throughout the day. If CADS cannot be installed in all classrooms used by students who require amplification, a personal FM system that can move with the student may be more appropriate.

◆ Infrared Technology

Over the last decade, infrared CADS has increased rapidly in popularity among audiologists and educators. In these systems, the acoustic signal from a microphone is frequency-modulated onto a carrier frequency, which is, in turn, amplitude-modulated by light-emitting diodes (LEDs) in the infrared spectrum. The infrared receiver uses photodetector diodes to pick up and convert the signal into electrical energy for delivery via loudspeaker.

Infrared light has a wavelength longer than that of visible light. Because light in this spectrum does not penetrate or bend around solid surfaces, infrared transmission requires line-of-sight communication between the transmitter and receiver to function. This means that the signal may drop out if a physical obstruction is placed in the signal path. However, it also means that a properly installed infrared system is not subject to interference from systems in nearby rooms—a significant potential advantage over FM transmission when multiple systems are in use within a single building.

Modern infrared CADS typically delivers a high-fidelity signal, contributing to the increasing popularity of this technology. Infrared offers other advantages as well: because the number of carrier frequencies is virtually unlimited, it is possible to have multiple microphones in use within a single room without one interfering with another. Many newer systems offer at least two microphones—one for use by the teacher and one as a pass-around microphone for children to use when asking and answering questions or participating in group activities.

Infrared technology does have some drawbacks. First, these systems historically have been more expensive than FM systems. The popularity of infrared technology has increased the number of infrared CADS manufacturers and narrowed this gap, but FM remains a less expensive option in most settings. Second, infrared is subject to interference from bright sunlight, making these systems inappropriate for highly sunlit rooms or outdoor use. More rarely, bright fluorescent light can interfere with infrared transmission. Finally, if multiple infrared emitters are required to ensure adequate signal coverage of a room (such as in a large room or one in which not every student can be seated with line-of-sight to a single emitter), the addition of supplementary emitters may complicate installation and increase cost.

◆ Analog Electromagnetic Induction Loops

Electromagnetic analog induction loop amplification systems are one of the oldest forms of room amplification, but are less commonly used with CADS compared with the technologies described previously. In a loop system, a microphone is connected (via hard wire or wirelessly) to an amplifier. The amplifier transmits the electrical signal from the microphone to a length of insulated copper wire encircling the room. The electrical current flowing through the wire creates an electromagnetic field that can be picked up by any device using a telecoil. A telecoil consists of a thin conductive wire wound around a ferrous metal core. When electricity passes through the wire, a magnetic field is created that can be picked up by the device containing the telecoil and converted into an acoustical signal (see **Fig. 6.2** for a description of a typical loop system).

Many hearing aids include a telecoil option, and separate telecoil receivers can be worn by individuals who do not have hearing aids. Incremental improvements have been made in analog inductance systems, making the newer systems somewhat less prone to

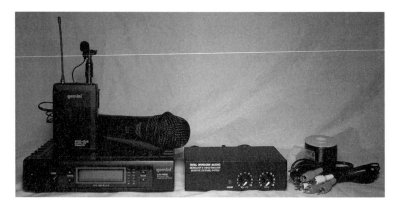

Fig. 6.2 Microloop III Dual FM (classroom-size loop system with wireless lavaliere teacher mike and hand-held wireless pass-around mike) from Oval Window Audio.

interference and better able to maintain consistent signal strength, but no major breakthroughs in technology are expected in the near term. A major improvement in analog inductance systems has come from a standard that specifies proper installation and performance rather than addressing it as an emerging technology. A new inductance loop standard published by the International Electrotechnical Commission (2006) specifies reference magnetic field strength levels and coverage as well as acceptable background SNR levels. Compliance with the standard should equalize the performance of analog inductance systems in terms of useful listening volume and frequency response. Inductance systems installed without regard to the standard may lead to unpredictable and possibly substandard performance.

Induction loop systems provide several potential advantages over other CADS options. First, they tend to be the least expensive of all forms of room amplification. A major reason for this lower cost is that receivers are not part of the induction loop system: the receiver is typically the listener's hearing aid or cochlear implant, or a separate telecoil-enabled receiver. Second, loop systems have few components and are simple to install both in new and existing rooms. Maintenance of induction loop systems tends to be simple, and replacement of the wire loop is generally inexpensive.

There are some significant limitations to induction loops as an option for CADS. The most obvious of these is that loop systems require each child in the classroom to have a telecoil-enabled hearing aid or loop receiver, making the signal more difficult to access by children without hearing loss or who do not use hearing aids regularly. Furthermore, each child's telecoil must be functional and sufficiently sensitive to pick up the looped signal. This requires the educational audiologist or child's own audiologist to be vigilant in maintaining a child's hearing aid(s) to ensure continual access to the signal in the classroom. Unfortunately, even many functional telecoils do not provide enough gain for the child to make use of the loop signal. Verification of the telecoil function in each receiver (hearing aid or separate) is therefore necessary prior to the use of loop technology.

Second, many hearing aids with a telecoil do not offer a microphone-plus-telecoil (M+T) option. Absence of the M+T option requires the child to choose between accessing the electrical signal via the telecoil, resulting in a loss of access to any signal to the microphone such as other children asking questions, and accessing the acoustic classroom signal and losing the benefit of the induction loop signal.

Third, the signal quality of a loop system varies as a function of the distance from the wire loop. That is, the farther away an individual moves from the induction loop, the poorer the signal received, which could lead to a loss of speech perception. For induction loop systems to be viable as CADS, the loop must be installed so that all children are seated near it. A further limitation here is that the strength of the electrical signal decreases as a function of loop size, so the larger loops necessary to encompass a large classroom may provide too weak a signal to assist all individuals in the room.

Finally, induction loop systems are subject to interference from several sources. Other electrical devices in the room that produce magnetic fields may create noise that is picked up by telecoils in the room. Two examples of interference sources are fluorescent lighting and unshielded electrical power lines, both of which generate a 60 Hz hum that may be heard on the telecoil circuit. Induction loops in nearby spaces may interfere with one another as well. Energy spillover from an induction loop may extend as far as 50 to 100 feet from the loop itself, meaning that listeners may hear signals from adjacent or other nearby looped rooms. The nature of induction loop systems is such that there is only one "channel" on which to broadcast, so the number of rooms appropriate for induction loops in a school may be limited.

◆ Hardwired and Wireless Public Address Systems

A less expensive but often much less effective alternative to CADS is the public address (PA) system. These systems typically include a microphone connected by a wire to a single-unit amplifier/loudspeaker, although some systems do employ wireless microphones or multiple speaker arrays. The relatively low cost and easy availability of these systems makes them attractive to school administrators attempting to provide amplification on a budget, and there is limited evidence that they may be effective for this purpose in certain populations, such as for individuals with cognitive declines or physical disabilities (Weinstein & Amsel, 1986).

However, these systems have significant disadvantages compared with systems designed for the specific purpose of providing amplification in the classroom. Most important, public address systems are not rated as medical devices by the Food and Drug Administration (FDA), so there are no federal standards for these units' electroacoustic characteristics, including gain, frequency response, and distortion. A PA system therefore should be expected to provide a lower-quality signal than FDA-approved CADS, particularly inexpensive off-the-shelf PA devices. Second, single-speaker systems are unlikely to provide a uniform signal throughout the classroom, which is a major goal in the installation of any CADS. Third, hardwired PA devices restrict the movement of the teacher to a point near the amplifier/loudspeaker and limit the use of a pass-around microphone.

Tables 6.1, 6.2, 6.3, 6.4, and **6.5** detail some of the potential advantages and disadvantages of signal transmission options available in CADS. Also included in the tables are lists of manufacturers and distributors for each technology type. It should be noted that these lists are intended to be representative rather than comprehensive. They do not imply endorsement of these companies or non-endorsement of unlisted companies.

◆ Emerging CADS Technology

The technology used in CADS is evolving and promises to further improve the SNR and quality of the sound received by every student in the classroom. While small improvements in the technologies already described will continue, this section will focus on cutting-edge technologies that may already be available in CADS products by some manufacturers, and some technologies that may become widely available in the near future.

Table 6.1 Potential Advantages and Disadvantages of Sound-Field FM CADS, with Selected Manufacturers and Distributors

Advantages	Disadvantages	Manufacturers and Distributors
Because line-of-sight is not needed, these systems typically experience no signal dropout	Finite number of clear carrier frequencies for transmission may limit the number of FM units usable in a single school	Centrum Sound Systems (www.centrumsound.com)
Typically less expensive than other wireless technologies, such as infrared	Transmissions on adjacent frequency bands may spill over or result in loss of fidelity	Comtek (www.comtek.com) Phonak Hearing Systems (www.phonak.com) Phonic Ear (www.phonicear.com)
Large number of manufacturers and systems means flexibility with regard to number of loudspeakers, installation options, etc.	Interference may result from powerful FM broadcasters, including radio stations and police/ emergency services	Lifeline Audio Video Technologies (www.lifelineav.com) Sennheiser Electronics (www.sennheiserusa.com)
	Use of multiple microphones within a single system may deplete available carrier frequencies	TeachLogic (www.teachlogic.com) Telex (www.telex.com)

◆ Loudspeakers

The goals in the installation of any CADS are to make the sound approximately uniform in volume throughout the room, minimize feedback, minimize late reflections, and amplify transparently. That is, it should not be obvious that the teacher's voice is being amplified. The loudspeakers conventionally used in CADS (and virtually all loudspeaker designs) are considered a spherical-wave source. Sound from a spherical-wave source radiates in three dimensions, like an expanding sphere or balloon: forward, left/right, and up/down. Spherical waves retain only one-fourth of their sound intensity with each doubling of distance from the source and often exhibit a non-uniform frequency response in a location other than directly in front of the source. This distribution of energy over an increasing area is heard as a substantial reduction in sound level as the listener moves away from the loudspeaker. Audiologists, of course, are familiar with this type of wave behavior and refer to it as the "inverse square law." Critics of the use of audio distribution

Table 6.2 Potential Advantages and Disadvantages of Infrared CADS, with Selected Manufacturers and Distributors

Advantages	Disadvantages	Manufacturers and Distributors
Unlimited number of possible carrier frequencies	Bright sunlight, fluorescent light, and other infrared sources may interfere with transmission	Atlas Sound (www.atlassound.com)
Multiple microphone use possible		Audio Enhancement (www.audioenhancement.com)
Infrared light cannot penetrate solid walls, which limits interference from adjacent classroom systems	Requires line-of-sight between transmitter and all receivers	Lifeline Audio Video Technologies (www.lifelineav.com)
	May be prone to signal dropout due to obstructions in the room, such as moving students	LightSpeed Technologies (www.lightspeed-tek.com)
		PhonicEar (www.phonicear.com)
	Typically more expensive than FM systems	Sennheiser Electronics (www.sennheiserusa.com)
	Need for multiple emitters may increase cost and complicate installation	SMART (www.smarttech.com)
		TeachLogic (www.teachlogic.com)

systems in classrooms cite this rapid reduction in sound intensity and the fact that the waves radiate in many directions as a potential source for the generation of late reflection patterns. Late reflections, also called reverberation, add masking and distortion to speech signals and are not desirable. In systems with this type of loudspeaker design, to make up for the loss of intensity as a function of distance and to limit the generation of late reflection patterns, multiple loudspeakers (or distributed sound systems) are typically used, with each student placed close to a loudspeaker so that direct sound predominates and the influence of late reverberation is minimized. A well-designed classroom audio distribution system can greatly improve the classroom sound quality, but it is difficult to overcome the inherent limitations of a spherical-wave sound source.

To improve on the limitations of a spherical-wave sound source, alternative types of loudspeaker designs have recently made their way into audio distribution systems. One such design is considered a cylindrical-wave source. A cylindrical-wave source is shaped like

Table 6.3 Potential Advantages and Disadvantages of Electromagnetic Induction Loop CADS, with Selected Manufacturers and Distributors

Advantages	Disadvantages	Manufacturers and Distributors
For students who have hearing aids with telecoils, no separate receiver or headset is required to access the signal	Requires users to have hearing aids/cochlear implants with a telecoil option or a separate telecoil-enabled receiver to access the signal	American Loop Services (www.americanloops.com)
Signal is filtered by the students' hearing aids, to be optimized for each individual	Hearing aid/cochlear implant users without an M+T option must choose either the acoustic or electro-magnetic signal for listening	Ampetronic/Assistive Audio (www.ampetronic.com or www.assistiveaudio.com)
Operates on a universal frequency	Signal quality (and therefore speech recognition) decreases as a function of distance from the induction loop	Anchor Audio (www.anchoraudio.com)
	Spillover may result when more than one loop is used in adjacent or other nearby rooms	Assistive Hearing Systems (www.assistivehearingsystems.com)
		Complete Hearing Solutions (www.completehearingonline.com)
		Contacta (www.contactainc.com)
		Hearing Loop Systems (www.hearingloopsystems.com)
		inLoop (www.inloop.tv)
		Loop America (www.loopamerica.com)
		Oval Window Audio (www.ovalwindowaudio.com)
		Phonic Ear (www.phonicear.com)

a vertical line or pole. Cylindrical sound waves radiate in only two dimensions—forward and to the right/left, but not up/down. Cylindrical waves do not lose intensity with distance as fast as spherical waves; rather, they lose only half their intensity with each doubling of distance. Listeners experience this reduction of sound intensity with distance as modest compared with a spherical-wave source. Because sound is radiated in only two dimensions, not as many surfaces are energized and so not as many late reflection patterns are created to degrade speech as with a spherical-wave source.

Table 6.4 Potential Advantages and Disadvantages of Hardwired and Wireless Public Address Systems, with Selected Manufacturers and Distributors

Advantages	Disadvantages	Manufacturers and Distributors
Many PA systems are portable single-unit systems that may be used in more than one classroom during the day Typically less expensive than FM or infrared systems	Public address systems generally are not engineered for classroom use and may deliver an inferior signal Wired connection limits movement of the teacher or speaker	Anchor Audio (www.anchoraudio.com) Audio Enhancement (www.audioenhancement.com) Centrum Sound Systems (www.centrumsound.com) Phonic Ear (www.phonicear.com)

Table 6.5 Potential Advantages and Disadvantages of Bluetooth CADS, with Selected Manufacturers and Distributors

Advantages	Disadvantages	Manufacturers and Distributors
Encryption may allow for secure transmission, limiting interference from nearby systems Synchronization between Bluetooth transmitters and receivers is simple and typically quick Advances in Bluetooth compatibility among hearing aids may allow direct access to CADS through this technology for children with aided hearing loss	At this writing, no Bluetooth CADS are yet commercially available; this technology is expected to become available in the near future Bluetooth devices typically have a high rate of power drain, which may limit wireless use throughout the school day	No manufacturers of Bluetooth CADS could be identified at the time of this writing

Other newer loudspeaker designs also are aimed at reducing the loss of intensity with distance, the variation of frequency response, and the generation of late reflection patterns. In addition to the cylindrical design, flat panel, bending wave technologies and plane wave sources are being refined. The application of these speaker advances to classroom audio distribution systems may further enhance the effectiveness of these systems (Eargle, 2010).

◆ Digital Transmission Technology

Recently, digital transmission has been incorporated into CADS to overcome problems of interference, limited channel bandwidth, and signal dead spots. Digital modulation, introduced by one manufacturer (H. Mulder, personal communication, 2011), uses the 2.4 GHz frequency band to package digitized audio signals into short digital bursts of code that are broadcast on different channels. Designed to frequency-hop among the channels between 2.4 and 2.485 GHz, systems using this technology avoid the problem of limited channel availability due to channel interference common to FM transmission schemes. Due to the digitization of the signal, advanced signal processing can be applied, such as error correction in the transmission and dynamic maintenance of desirable SNRs. Because of these and other advantages, we should see increasing use of digital transmission in future CADS.

◆ Bluetooth Technology

Bluetooth is a proprietary open wireless technology standard for exchanging data over short distances using short-wavelength radio transmissions in the ISM (Industry, Scientific, Medical) band from 2400 to 2480 MHz. Fixed and mobile devices may employ Bluetooth to create personal area networks (PANs) with high levels of security. Bluetooth streaming has enjoyed some application in connecting cell phones and hearing aids. While it has potential in the CADS area, there are no current commercial CADS offerings using this technology. It should also be noted that some CADS varieties that transmit using other methods do employ Bluetooth communications to interface with devices like media players.

◆ Digital Inductance Transmission Technology

Digital inductance transmission is different from the analog inductance systems covered earlier. The analog audio signal from the microphone is transformed into a digital stream by an analog-to-digital converter. The digital data are then coded and modulated onto an inductive carrier frequency in the lower megahertz range. This coded and modulated signal is fed into a loop of wire that generates a magnetic field. The field is received by a special coil and is demodulated and decoded to retrieve the transmitted digitized signal. The digital signal is then converted back into an analog signal by a digital-to-analog converter and processed as an analog signal. In order for this to work, the transmitter and receiver need to use the same carrier frequency, the same modulation, and same protocol to code/decode the audio signal. Therefore, digital inductance is usually not compatible between manufacturers (E. Dijkstra, personal communication, 2011).

Digital inductance loop technology promises less interference, a wider frequency band, and a more consistent signal. The downside is that the signal cannot be received by the typical analog telecoil found in modern hearing aids, and so the technology does not enjoy universal compatibility. While some manufacturers may include coils for both analog and digital inductance in their hearing aids, the simplicity, low cost, and universal applicability of analog inductance systems argues against the prospect of widespread use of digital inductance technology, at least in the near future.

◆ Automatic Noise Compensation Technology

The background noise levels in classrooms fluctuate (Blair, 1977; Larsen & Blair, 2008) from −7 to +15 as a function of classroom activity. An SNR of +15 dB throughout the classroom is generally considered desirable for classroom instruction (ANSI, 2010), so attainment of SNR with fluctuating background noise has been a challenge for CADS. Attempts to equalize the SNR throughout the room have included use of multiple loudspeakers throughout the room, student placement closer to speakers, and use of new speaker designs (Crandell, Smaldino, & Flexer, 2005; Smaldino, 2011). As early as 2000, Lederman, DeConde Johnson, Crandell, and Smaldino (2000) reported on the development of a "Smart Speaker" system that would monitor background noise levels and automatically adjust the SNR to a favorable level. While this system did not catch on with the manufacturers of CADS at the time, a new CADS product has recently been introduced that maintains a favorable SNR in the classroom using the latest in smart electronics (H. Mulder, personal communication, 2011). Maintenance of a favorable SNR amidst the dynamically changing background noise level of a classroom is very desirable, and it is expected that other manufacturers will incorporate this technology in the near future.

References

American National Standards Institute (ANSI) (2010). *Acoustical performance criteria, design requirements, and guidelines for schools, Part 1: Permanent schools* (ANSI S12.60-2010/Part 1). New York, NY: Acoustical Society of America.

Blair, J. C. (1977). Effects of amplification, speechreading, and classroom environments on reception of speech. *Volta Review, 79*(7), 443–449.

Crandell, C. C., Smaldino, J. J., & Flexer, C. (Eds.). (2005) *Sound field amplification: Applications to speech perception and classroom acoustics* (2nd Ed., pp. 72–111). Clifton Park, NY: Delmar Cengage Learning.

Eargle, J. (2010). *Loudspeaker handbook* (2nd Ed.). New York, NY: Springer.

Edwards, D., & Fuen, L. (2005). A formative evaluation of sound-field amplification system across several grade levels in four schools. *Journal of Educational Audiology, 12,* 59–66.

Iglehart, F. (2004, June). Speech perception by students with cochlear implants using sound-field systems in classrooms. *American Journal of Audiology, 13*(1), 62–72.

International Electrotechnical Commission. (2006), IEC 60118–4. *Inductance loop standard.* Geneva: International Electrotechnical Commission.

Larsen, J. B., & Blair, J. C. (2008, October). The effect of classroom amplification on the signal-to-noise ratio in classrooms while class is in session. *Language, Speech, and Hearing Services in Schools, 39*(4), 451–460.

Lederman, N., DeConde Johnson, C., Crandell, C. C., & Smaldino, J. J. (2000). The development and validation of an "intelligent" classroom sound field frequency modulation (FM) system. *Journal of Educational Audiology, 7,* 37–42.

Lewis, D. E. (1991). FM systems and assistive devices: Selection and evaluation. In J. Feigin & P. G. Stelmachowicz (Eds.), *Pediatric amplification* (pp. 139–152). Omaha, NE: Boys Town National Research Hospital.

Rosenberg, G. G. (2005). Sound field amplification: A comprehensive literature review. In C. C. Crandell, J. J. Smaldino, & C. Flexer (Eds.), *Sound field amplification: Applications to speech perception and classroom acoustics* (2nd Ed., pp. 72–111). Clifton Park, NY: Delmar Cengage Learning.

Rosenberg, G. G., Blake-Rahter, P., Heavner, J., Allen, L., Redmond, B., Phillips, J., et al. (1999). Improving classroom acoustics (ICA): A three-year FM sound field classroom amplification study. *Journal of Educational Audiology, 7,* 8–28.

Ryan, S. (2009, April). The effects of a sound-field amplification system on managerial time in middle school physical education settings. *Language, Speech, and Hearing Services in Schools, 40*(2), 131–137.

Sapienza, C. M., Crandell, C. C., & Curtis, B. (1999, September). Effects of sound-field frequency modulation amplification on reducing teachers' sound pressure level in the classroom. *Journal of Voice, 13*(3), 375–381.

Sarff, L. (1981). An innovative use of free-field amplification in classrooms. In R. Roeser & M. Downs (Eds.), *Auditory disorders in school children* (pp. 263–272). New York: Thieme-Stratton.

Smaldino, J. J. (2011). New developments in classroom acoustics and amplification. *Audiology Today, 23*(1), 30–36.

Weinstein, B. E., & Amsel, L. (1986). Hearing loss and senile dementia in the institutionalized elderly. *Clinical Gerontologist, 4,* 3–15.

Wilson, W. J., Marinac, J., Pitty, K., & Burrows, C. (2011, October). The use of sound-field amplification devices in different types of classrooms. *Language, Speech, and Hearing Services in Schools, 42*(4), 395–407.

7

Best Practices: AAA Clinical Practice Guidelines for Hearing Assistance Technology

Cheryl DeConde Johnson

Hearing assistance technology (HAT) closes the gap between audibility and understanding. Consequently, every user of hearing instruments as well as other listeners who need or want to enhance their listening experience should be considered candidates for HAT. The American Academy of Audiology's Clinical Practice Guidelines for Remote Microphone Hearing Assistance Technologies for Children and Youth Birth to 21 Years (American Academy of Audiology, 2008) provides a rationale and comprehensive protocol for these devices. The protocol contains a core statement that addresses the complex process of HAT selection, fitting, and management plus supplements that outline procedures for fitting and verification of ear-level FM (Supplement A) and classroom audio distribution systems (CADS) (Supplement B). A third supplement, for personal neck loops, is under development. The core statement was designed to provide general information pertinent to HAT. Each supplement's procedures are technology dependent, so the supplements are to be revised by the AAA HAT Task Force as technologies evolve. Professional practice standards, in addition to describing a profession's recommendations for practice, are important for justifying practices with administrators, funding agencies, and consumers. The HAT document contents are outlined in **Table 7.1**.

This chapter will highlight important facets of the guidelines, including verification procedures recommended in Supplement B for selection and fitting of CADS. It is recommended that readers who are involved in HAT review and maintain a current version of the guidelines and the supplements. Furthermore, the HAT guidelines cite evidence for statements and recommendations that are made.

Table 7.1 Contents of Clinical Practice Guidelines for Remote Microphone Hearing Assistance Technologies for Children and Youth Birth to 21 Years

1. Introduction
2. Regulatory Considerations
3. Personnel Qualifications
4. Equipment and Space Requirements
5. Remote Microphone HAT Candidacy, Implementation and Device Selection Considerations
6. Fitting and Verification Procedures
7. Implementation and Validation Procedures
8. References
9. Appendices
10. Supplements

◆ Regulatory Considerations

Knowledge of regulations that support the implementation of HAT is necessary in advocating with administrative and funding entities. The primary regulations that impact HAT are contained in the Individuals with Disabilities Education Act (IDEA), the Rehabilitation Act of 1973, and the Americans with Disabilities Act (ADA).

1. IDEA provides for individual evaluation for the HAT device, and for maintenance and management of the use of the device when the Individual Education Program (IEP) or Individual Family Service Plan (IFSP) team determines that the HAT device is necessary for the child or youth to receive a free and appropriate public education (FAPE). Federal and state funding supports the provision of HAT in public schools.

2. Section 504 of the Rehabilitation Act requires reasonable accommodations for persons of all ages with disabilities in any facility or by any entity that receives public funds. The accommodations for Section 504 are delineated for each individual in a 504 Plan. Accommodations are paid for by the responsible entity.

3. ADA requires accommodations for persons with disabilities in all public places. Accommodations are paid for by the responsible entity.

The pertinent regulations within these laws are summarized in **Table 7.2**. Appendix 7.1 contains the full IDEA citations noted in **Table 7.2**.

◆ Overview of Core Statement

The HAT guidelines make several important points regarding fitting of HAT, including:

1. Audiologists are the professionals singularly qualified to select and fit all forms of amplification equipment for children and youth, including HAT.
2. Audiologists fitting HAT should have the expertise and test equipment necessary to complete all aspects of the device selection, evaluation, and verification procedures.

In addition, audiologists should be mindful of each step in the HAT process, recognizing that HAT involves much more than just fitting a device to a child or youth.

The purpose of HAT is to improve access to the talker by minimizing the harmful effects of noise, distance, and reverberation. The HAT guidelines target three wireless options and three listening groups. The wireless options are:

1. Personal devices in which the speech signal is processed and transmitted to a hearing aid, cochlear implant, bone conductive device, or other personal hearing device;
2. Wide area and targeted area CADS, in which the signal is sent to one or more strategically positioned loudspeakers;
3. Personal induction loop technology, in which the speech signal is sent to a personal hearing instrument via a magnetic signal generated by a loop of wire or other inductor.

The three listening groups include:

1. Children and youth with hearing loss who are actual or potential hearing aid users;
2. Children and youth with cochlear implants and bone conduction hearing devices;
3. Children and youth with normal hearing sensitivity who have special listening requirements.

The guidelines are organized into five steps, which are illustrated in **Fig. 7.1.**

Table 7.2 Summary of IDEA, Section 504, and ADA

Law/Regulation	Main Themes	Regulatory Authority

IDEA: Individuals with Disabilities Education Act (IDEA, 2004), http://idea.ed.gov	• Free and appropriate public education (FAPE)
	• Education in the least restrictive environment (LRE)
	• Individual education program (IEP), Part B
	• Individual family service plan (IFSP), Part C
	• Regulations pertaining to the use of hearing instruments and HAT
	
	  34 CFR 300.34(c)(1): Definition of Audiology (Part B)
	  34 CFR 303.13(b)(2): Definition of Audiology (Part C)
	  34 CFR 300.5-6, 34 CFR 303.13(b)(1)(i): Assistive Technology and Assistive Technology Services (Part B and Part C)
	  34 CFR 300.105(a)(2): Assistive Technology Used at Home or Other Settings
	  34 CFR 300.324(2)(iv): Development, Review, and Revision of IEP, Consideration of Special Factors
		Office of Special Education Programs, Office of Special Education and Rehabilitative Services, U.S. Department of Education.

Section 504 (Rehabilitation Act, 1973), http://www.ed.gov/about/offices/list/ocr/docs/edlite-FAPE504.html Subpart A: General Provisions Subpart B: Employment Practices Subpart C: Program Accessibility Subpart D: Preschool, Elementary, and Secondary Education	School age: free and appropriate public education (FAPE). Other populations: all employers, schools and educational programs, nursing homes, mental health centers, and human services programs that receive or benefit from federal financial assistance. Under Section 504, any qualified individual with a disability has the right to a reasonable accommodation, such as services or aids, to help that individual participate in the programs or jobs offered by the federally funded employer, school, or other organization.	Office for Civil Rights (OCR), U. S. Department of Education

Subpart E: Post-Secondary Setting Subpart F: Health, Welfare, and Social Services Subpart G: Procedures	Post-secondary: • Appropriate academic adjustments as necessary to ensure that it does not discriminate on the basis of disability. If the post-secondary school provides housing to non-disabled students, it must provide comparable convenient and accessible housing to students with disabilities at the same cost. • Program does not have to make modifications that would fundamentally alter the nature of a service, program, or activity or would result in undue financial or administrative burdens.	
ADA: Americans with Disabilities Act • Title II: all services, programs, and activities provided to the public by state and local governments, including state-operated schools, colleges, and universities • Title III: places of public accommodation (businesses and nonprofit agencies that serve the public) and "commercial facilities" (other businesses), including private schools, colleges, and universities	Prohibits discrimination on the basis of disability; sections include (responsible agency in parentheses): • Employment (Equal Employment Opportunity Center) • Public Transportation (U.S. Department of Transportation) • Telephone Relay Service (Federal Communications Commission) • Design Guidelines (U.S. Access Board) • Education (U.S. Department of Education) • Health Care (U.S. Department of Health and Human Services) • Labor (U.S. Department of Labor) • Housing (U.S. Department of Housing and Urban Development) • Parks and Recreation (U.S. Department of the Interior) • Agriculture (U.S. Department of Agriculture)	Education: Office for Civil Rights (OCR) in the U.S. Department of Education All other areas: U.S. Department of Justice, Civil Rights Division, Disability Rights Section *A Guide to Disability Rights Law* (September 2005), http://www.ada.gov/publicat.htm#Anchor-14210

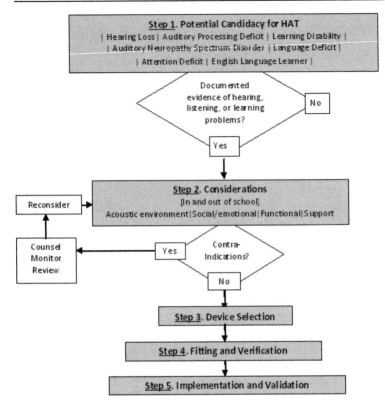

Fig. 7.1 HAT candidacy, device selection, and implementation process.

◆ Candidacy, Implementation, and Device Selection Considerations

Candidacy

As described in the first step, candidacy involves the consideration of children and youth with hearing loss as well as other groups who are often at risk for listening problems and who might benefit from improved auditory access to the talker. If there is any documented evidence of hearing, listening, or learning problems, whether in school or out of school (e.g., home, community), the process should move to step 2, where additional important issues are addressed prior to HAT implementation. These include whether HAT is needed to improve the acoustical environment; whether HAT will improve the developmental or academic functioning of the child or youth; and, most important, critical social-emotional areas, including motivation, attention and fatigue, self-image, self-advocacy, social acceptance, classroom culture, and family support. As children age, the decision of whether to recommend HAT must weigh the acoustic and listening benefits along with the social-emotional ability of the child to accept and use the device. When a child is not ready, or when there is not a current need based on the functional or acoustical environmental status, the audiologist and school team must provide counseling for the student, monitor the situation, and review and reconsider the use of HAT as the situation changes.

Device Selection

Once candidacy has been established, the audiologist should proceed to step 3, device selection. Audiological, developmental, listening environment (in school and out of school), and technology considerations are described in the guidelines and summarized along with implementation decisions in **Fig. 7.2**. Default HAT fitting arrangements recommended for each listening group are described in **Table 7.3**. IDEA is the primary HAT

Table 7.3 Default HAT Fitting Arrangements Based on Listening Needs*

Group	Default Fitting Arrangement
Group 1: children and youth with hearing loss who are actual or potential hearing aid users	Bilateral ear-level wireless technology
Group 2: children and youth with cochlear implants or bone conduction hearing devices	Headband-anchored: ear-level wireless technology Bone-anchored: no default HAT arrangement**
Group 3: children and youth with normal hearing sensitivity who have special listening requirements	No default HAT arrangement

*Style and fitting considerations are based on hearing status; degree, configuration, and stability of loss; current use of hearing technology; and any other special situations that are present.
**While children with bone-anchored hearing devices would benefit from enhanced SNRs, there is no research to support a specific arrangement.

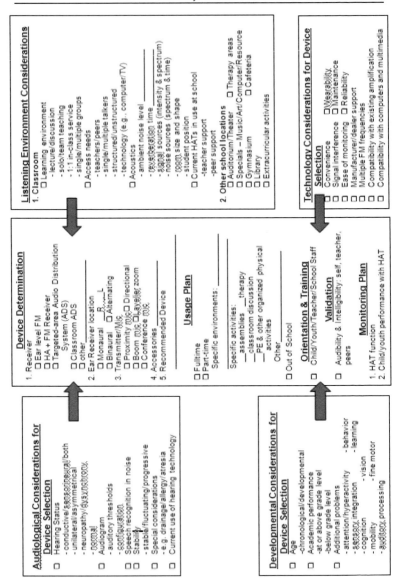

Fig. 7.2 HAT in-school implementation plan.

funding source for school-age children who are eligible for special education; 504 and ADA funding should be explored for others, and private sources may be needed for private schools and other non-public entities (e.g., churches, clubs). FM or assistive technology loan banks may be operated by some state education programs. Once all components of the selection process have been considered, a HAT device, including receiver, transmitter, and accessories, is selected.

Fitting and Verification

The HAT guidelines detail specific procedures for fitting and verifying the selected device (step 4) for both ear-level FM (Supplement A) and CADS (Supplement B). Both supplements include fitting and verification worksheets; an illustrated version of Supplement A is available on DVD through AAA. CADS fitting and verification recommendations are discussed in this chapter, and specific examples are provided in Chapter 8 of this handbook. Regardless of the device selected, the HAT guidelines recommend the following fitting goals based on best practices unless individual testing indicates otherwise:

1. Audibility and intelligibility
   a. Speech recognition that is commensurate with performance in ideal listening conditions.
   b. Full audibility of self and others.
   c. Reduced effects of distance, noise, and reverberation.
2. Preferred practice to accomplish full audibility
   a. Consistent signal from the talker regardless of head movement.
   b. Technology that will be worn consistently by the individual, parent, and/or teacher.
   c. Technology that will provide full audibility according to listener group:
      • *Group 1. Children and youth with hearing loss who are actual or potential hearing aid users:* Bilateral ear-level wireless technology and requiring the fewest equipment adjustments.
      • *Group 2. Children and youth with cochlear implants or bone-conduction hearing devices:* Bilateral wireless technology.

- *Group 3. Children and youth with normal hearing sensitivity who have special listening requirements:* There is no default HAT arrangement for this population.

Implementation and Validation

Recommendations for HAT use are effective only if they are implemented appropriately. Therefore, special attention needs to be given to ensure that sufficient orientation, training, and monitoring are provided to support appropriate implementation of HAT devices. A usage plan should specify the full- or part-time use recommendations as well as considerations for use outside of school. Step 5 of the HAT guidelines details recommendations for these areas as well as validation procedures. The purpose of validation is to ensure that the selected device is providing the expected outcomes for the child or youth. Validation procedures for HAT include a combination of self-assessments, observation questionnaires, and evaluation. Once validation is confirmed, the final component of HAT is development of a monitoring plan to identify who is responsible for checking the functionality of the device, when, how often, what procedures will be used, and what will happen when the device malfunctions. Each of these implementation and validation procedures is required under IDEA for eligible children and youth (see Appendix 7.1). **Fig. 7.2** summarizes the steps from selection considerations to the monitoring plan.

CADS Considerations

According to Supplement B of the AAA HAT guidelines, the purpose of CADS is to maintain a consistent speech-to-noise (S/N) ratio throughout a classroom or listening space. CADS is often necessary to overcome the effects of loud noise sources, such as ventilation systems. However, CADS should not be used as a remedy for inadequate acoustical treatment of the learning environment. Therefore, in considering whether CADS is appropriate for a classroom, acoustical measurements must be conducted as a first step. Chapter 4 of this handbook, and particularly Appendix 4.1, discuss procedures for observation and measurement of classroom acoustics.

The CADS selection and fitting guidelines identify three groups of potential candidates: children and youth with no special listening requirements; children and youth with hearing loss who use hearing aids, cochlear implants, or bone conduction devices who may be using a personal FM; and children and youth with normal hearing sensitivity who have special listening requirements and who may be using a personal FM. Set-up procedures for loudspeaker placement, intensity levels, frequency response, and feedback are addressed. Verification measures are described for each of the three groups that address "real room" and behavioral procedures.

Compatibility with personal FM systems is an important consideration with the use of CADS. Audiologists have two signal transmission options: parallel and sequential signal processing. In parallel signal transmission, the talker wears the microphone/transmitters for both the personal FM system and the CADS, delivering signals independently to each system. In sequential processing, the talker wears the FM microphone/transmitter sending the signal to the CADS amplifier via the FM receiver that is connected to the audio input port. While this method delivers the talker signal to both the personal FM receiver and the CADS, possible electroacoustic variations in the CADS signal may occur. When considering a sequential processing design, the audiologist must determine whether there is interference between the systems and under what conditions—and then, after initial compatibility is established, whether subsequent adjustments to the first system degrade the signal of the second system. The audiologist also needs to determine the arrangement that the teacher can best manage while maintaining signal integrity. Another fitting option is selecting an FM system that is designed to incorporate both personal FM and CADS signal transmission. In this parallel mode, the signal is processed independently for each receiver, maintaining the integrity of each signal.

◆ Summary

Effective HAT implementation requires a comprehensive process that ensures audibility of self and others, reduces effects of distance, noise, and reverberation, and closes the gap between audibility and intelligibility. Furthermore, the process must recognize the importance of the consumer as well as the support that is required for appropriate and consistent implementation. **Table 7.4** describes strategies recommended by educational audiologists to assist with implementation of the HAT guidelines in the schools.

Table 7.4 Strategies for Implementing the AAA HAT Guidelines in Schools

Area	Strategies
1. Personnel qualifications	• Incorporate administrators (principals) into trainings so they understand and can implement requirements of standards • Enlist support of professional colleagues (teachers of DHH students, SLPs) to adhere to professional scope of practice and state licensure requirements • Contract with a clinical audiologist • Find an audiologist who can perform testing for minimal cost • Work with clinical audiologists regarding the procedures that are needed • Adhere to scope of practice standards
2. Equipment and space requirements	• Partner with clinical audiologists to share equipment and information • Have a central location with a sound booth for testing • Make nice with school staff, especially custodians, to garner space • Enlist resources for transportation • Test Real-Ear on site • Work closely with private/clinical audiologists (see Chapter 9 of this handbook) • Obtain information and implement measurements for room reverberation • Contract for evaluations • Renovate school or classroom for a sound booth • Tap into PTA, NCLB, and IDEA for funds • Work with funders (administrators) on guidelines regarding implementation • Create a loaner bank for equipment (e.g., Audioscan) • Rent from equipment providers
3. Candidacy, implementation, and device selection	• Look at regulatory issues in your state related to *who* can select HAT • Try to have good working relationships with clinical audiologists and physicians (see Chapter 9 of this handbook) • Cultivate parent and student education and support • Use YouTube training videos, Web sites, DVDs, PowerPoint presentations, SmartBoards • Provide continuing education for audiologists to encourage wide knowledge base • Develop protocol for functional testing to identify need for HAT (written procedures) (see Chapter 8 of this handbook) • Use questionnaires, DHH teacher assessments, SIFTER (see Chapter 8 of this handbook)

	• Follow written guidelines, e.g., target candidates (students with HL, cochlear implants, some LD, some CAPD) • Use the IEP process • Look at academic potential vs. performance—how to qualify for IEP and FM • Look at audiogram, academic, state testing, inventories, pre- and post-tests • Test for speech-in-noise performance; use BKB-SIN and FLE with and without HA and FM • Use pre- and post-trials to provide more objective criteria • Consider equipment warranties in HAT selection
4. Fitting and verification procedures	• Secure more concise information from manufacturers or AAA about verification procedures as technology changes • Develop a protocol for functional testing • Extend contractual services to add days before school starts to get FMs fitted • Use previous year's personal FM system fitting until schedule permits time to recheck • Contract with clinical audiologist to perform procedures • Seek public education or other funding • Secure Real-Ear testing equipment • AuD students to assist with procedures • Maintain communication with dispensing audiologist
5. Implementation and validation	• Make sure students understand and acknowledge the benefit of their technology. • Help students be "the boss" of their technology • Create "leave-behind" materials for teachers that are visual and easy to understand • Ensure that HAT is in the IEP and educate parents as advocates • Ensure that the school-based audiologist has the time and resources to perform validation and training • Assist clinical audiologist with performing validation procedures • Use questionnaires completed by teachers (e.g., LIFE, pre- and post-FM protocol, FLE, CHILD, IT-MAIS, SIFTER) • Conduct a schoolwide in-service at faculty meetings (use HL simulation and other real-world activities) • Train teachers, SLPs, or nurse to do daily checks • Provide DVDs for training on questionnaires • Provide education for parents • Ensure that these procedures are done as required by IDEA • Perform HA and FM validation at the same time • Provide in-service for school personnel to assist with validation

◆ Appendix 7.1
IDEA Regulations That Impact Provision of HAT

Part B. Definition of Audiology (34 CFR 300.34(c)(1))

Audiology includes

(i) Identification of children with hearing loss;

(ii) Determination of the range, nature, and degree of hearing loss, including referral for medical or other professional attention for the habilitation of hearing;

(iii) Provision of habilitation activities, such as language habilitation, auditory training, speech reading (lipreading), hearing evaluation, and speech conservation;

(iv) Creation and administration of programs for prevention of hearing loss;

(v) Counseling and guidance of children, parents, and teachers regarding hearing loss; and

(vi) Determination of children's needs for group and individual amplification, selecting and fitting an appropriate aid, and evaluating the effectiveness of amplification.

Part C. Definition of Audiology (34 CFR 303.13(b)(2) (2011))

Audiology services include

(i) Identification of children with auditory impairments, using at-risk criteria and appropriate audiological screening techniques;

(ii) Determination of the range, nature, and degree of hearing loss and communication functions, by use of audiologic evaluation procedures;

(iii) Referral for medical and other services necessary for the habilitation or rehabilitation of an infant or toddler with a disability who has an auditory impairment;

(iv) Provision of auditory training, aural rehabilitation, speech reading and listening devices, orientation and training, and other services;

(v) Provision of services for the prevention of hearing loss; and

(vi) Determination of the child's need for individual amplification, including selecting, fitting, and dispensing of appropriate listening and vibrotactile devices, and evaluating the effectiveness of those devices.

Assistive Technology (300.105(a)(2))

On a case-by-case basis, the use of school-purchased assistive technology devices in a child's home or in other settings is required if the child's IEP team determines that the child needs access to those devices to receive FAPE.

Part B. Development, Review, and Revision of IEP: Consideration of Special Factors (34 CFR 300.324(2)(iv))

The IEP team must

(iv) Consider the communication needs of the child, and in the case of a child who is deaf or hard of hearing, consider the child's language and communication needs, opportunities for direct communications with peers and professional personnel in the child's language and communication mode, academic level, and full range of needs, including opportunities for direct instruction in the child's language and communication mode;

(v) Consider whether the child requires assistive technology devices and services

Assistive Technology
Part B (34 CFR 300.5–.6)
Part C (34 CFR 303.13(b)(1))

Assistive technology device means any item, piece of equipment, or product system, whether acquired commercially off the shelf, modified, or customized, that is used to increase, maintain, or improve the functional capabilities of children with disabilities. The term does not include a medical device that is surgically implanted, or the replacement of such device.

Assistive technology service means any service that directly assists a child with a disability in the selection, acquisition, or use of an assistive technology device. The term includes

(a) The evaluation of the needs of a child with a disability, including a functional evaluation of the child in the child's customary environment;

(b) Purchasing, leasing, or otherwise providing for the acquisition of assistive technology devices by children with disabilities;

(c) Selecting, designing, fitting, customizing, adapting, applying, maintaining, repairing, or replacing assistive technology devices;

(d) Coordinating and using other therapies, interventions, or services with assistive technology devices, such as those associated with existing education and rehabilitation plans and programs;

(e) Training or technical assistance for a child with a disability or, if appropriate, that child's family; and

(f) Training or technical assistance for professionals (including individuals providing education or rehabilitation services), employers, or other individuals who provide services to, employ, or are otherwise substantially involved in the major life functions of children with disabilities.

References

American Academy of Audiology. (2008). Clinical practice guidelines: Remote microphone hearing assistance technologies for children and youth from birth to 21 years. Available at http://www.audiology.org

IDEA. (2004). Individuals with Disabilities Education Improvement Act of 2004, PL 108-446, 20 U.S.C. § 1400 et seq.

Rehabilitation Act. (1973). Section 504, 29 U.S.C. 794 et seq. *U.S. Statutes at Large, 87,* 335–394.

8 Approaches to Functional Verification of Classroom Accessibility

Karen L. Anderson

"Access denied is opportunity denied." (Howard, 2010)

Despite entering school with improved language and listening skills compared with students in prior decades, today's student with hearing loss continues to remain at a disadvantage when learning in a large group setting with fast-paced teacher and peer communications. Students with hearing loss are in situations every day in which they miss or mishear information and are expected to perform or respond without the advantage of having all of the information. The heart of learning differences for students with hearing loss is unequal or imperfect access to communication. Access is so important that the Individuals with Disabilities Education Act (IDEA, 2004) statute (20 USC 1400(c)(5)(H)) specifies "supporting the development and use of technology, including assistive technology devices and assistive technology services, to *maximize* accessibility for children with disabilities." Indeed, the "consideration of special factors" portion of IDEA (34 CFR 300.324(2)(iv)) states that the "IEP Team shall consider the communication needs of the child, and in the case of a child who is deaf or hard of hearing, consider the child's language and communication needs, [and] opportunities for direct communications with peers and professional personnel in the child's language and communication mode."

Access to curriculum and instruction in the classroom at the same level and rate as typically hearing peers is essential for academic growth for students with hearing loss. Technology has made it possible for most persons with hearing loss to hear and perceive speech in a manner approaching that of persons with typical hearing. Yet simply having the technology available does not inoculate the student against speech perception or understanding difficulties that could affect his or her attention and pace of learning over time. Only with equal acoustic access is the student able to receive *all* of the instruction and peer-to-peer communication that takes place within the classroom and in social situations. Equal access

105

also reflects the foundational belief that every student has the *right* to receive the same information as his or her class peers. Education builds understanding and critical thinking skills day by day, hour by hour, and minute by minute through information presented in school, formally, incidentally, and in all social situations. Access and communication skills are a gateway to an educated life. Allocation of appropriate technologies, accurate identification of student skills and communication correction issues, and student-focused advocacy to ensure that all needs are addressed are critical if true access to the general education curriculum is to be achieved.

All students learn by experiencing the world through their senses, and the auditory sense is the foundation of learning, especially early language learning. The speech signal is delivered at different intensities, at varying frequencies, and with dynamic changes in the rate and clarity of the words spoken. Other factors that affect speech understanding include background noise, reverberation, distance, attention, motivation, memory, linguistic complexity, and auditory processing ability. Hearing loss is complex in terms of its effect on perception and the resulting comprehension of speech. Thus, the focus of this chapter is not hearing loss per se, but the effect of the hearing loss on the student's ability to listen and subsequently learn and, especially, how the level of student acoustic access can be verified.

Defining a student's level of accessibility to verbal instruction is not straightforward. Accessibility relies on consideration of a variety of factors, including: speech audibility, speech understanding, challenges encountered in the classroom listening environment due to background noise and reverberation, and loudness of the teacher's voice above background noise. More specifically, we need to know how well the student is able to hear and understand louder (teacher voice) speech as well as soft speech, such as that of a peer answering a question from across the classroom. Therefore, functional verification of classroom intervention first requires that the student's level of accessibility to verbal instruction be identified.

◆ The First Question to Ask Is: How Well Can the Student Hear Speech?

1. The most relevant questions about a student's speech perception abilities are:

    a. How accurately can the student perceive speech when the speech signal is quiet (such as speech spoken at a distance)?

b. How accurately can the student perceive speech when the speech signal is loud (such as speech presented in close proximity)?

2. A line on an audiogram is far from an answer to the question "How well can this student hear speech?"

3. "Hearing speech" is not the same as hearing all of the specific sounds of all of the words. Speech sounds occur within a 30 dB range of intensity (*th* in "thaw" versus *oo* in "through"). Speech is dynamic and can change from soft speech to loud speech in a single sentence. The audiogram in **Fig. 8.1** represents various English speech sounds by their primary frequency (Hz) and intensity (dB) characteristics.

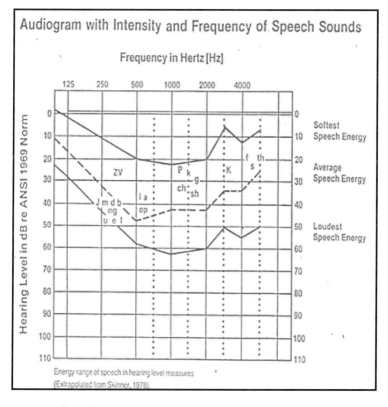

Fig. 8.1 This audiogram represents various English speech sounds by their primary frequency (Hz) and intensity (dB) characteristics.

◆ The Second Question to Ask Is: How do Students with Typical Hearing Perform in Background Noise?

Students with hearing loss compete with normally hearing students every school day. If we strive to supply students with hearing loss with equal access to verbal communication, then it is important to know how students with normal hearing perform, because this would be the goal for equal access. One study, cited in **Fig. 8.2**, looked at word recognition in quiet and noise for 126 children ages 3–17 years with typically developing hearing. Children repeated word lists at two different loudness levels: normal/loud conversa-

Results in %	Age 3-5 M - F	Age 6-8 M - F	Age 9+ M - F
Quiet 50 dB	98-98	98-98	99-96
Quiet 35 dB	95-96	97-98	98-96
50 dB @ +5 S/N	93-94	94-95	97-93
50 dB @ 0 S/N	91-92	91-93	95-93
35 dB @ 0 S/N	90-92	91-90	91-90

- 1999 data from Bodkin, Madell, and Rosenfeld
- 126 typically hearing children ages 3-17 years
- Listening at 35 and 50 dB HL.
- Age appropriate open set single word lists (NU-C, PBK, W-22)
- Competing noise = 4-talker babble.

The typical child performed at 90% or better = GOAL

Fig. 8.2 The typically developing child can perform at ~90 percent or better, even in high levels of background noise, when listening to soft speech (Bodkin, Madell, & Rosenfeld, 1999).

tional speech (50 dB HL) and soft or quiet voice loudness (35 dB HL). Age-appropriate open-set single-word lists were used, and the competing noise was four-talker speech babble. Word recognition scores (WR%) did not change significantly as listening became more difficult, regardless of gender or age.

The information in **Fig. 8.2** is very valuable for interpreting results of the Functional Listening Evaluation (FLE) (to download the entire FLE go to http://www.handsandvoices.org/pdf/func_eval.pdf). Unless the FLE is also performed on several typically hearing peers in exactly the same manner as it is performed on the student with hearing loss, there is no "standard" for comparison. Therefore, the findings of the study in **Fig. 8.2** can be used as the bar to which students with hearing loss are compared for communication access.

The Speech Intelligibility Index

Another way to represent a student's abilities to perceive speech is to consider his or her ability to hear the acoustic energy of speech sounds. This method changes the relative acoustic energy at each of the frequency bands into dots, which are then plotted on the Count-the-Dots Audiogram (Killion & Mueller, 2010). The more dots below the hearing threshold line, the more speech energy the student receives.

There is a much heavier distribution of dots between 1000 and 4000 Hz because this is the range that is most critical for discrimination of speech. Eleven percent of speech energy occurs above 4000 Hz, a frequency range most hearing instruments were not able to amplify until recent years. The Count-the-Dots Audiogram represents speech produced at an average loudness of 45 dB HL (conversational speech).

In a classroom setting, the teacher's voice is often at 50–60 dB HL. Students speaking quietly or from across a classroom have quiet speech energy at ~35 dB HL. Considering speech energy at a single speaker loudness will under-represent the listening challenges faced by students in a classroom setting. The exception to this is when a student uses a personal FM system to hear the teacher at a consistent loudness regardless of vocal loudness or direction. However, an FM system will not boost the loudness of classroom peers unless the teacher passes the FM microphone transmitter every time another student contributes to the class.

The *Speech Audibility Audiogram for Classroom Listening,* shown in **Fig. 8.3,** was developed by using the information from the Count-the-Dots Audiogram, which reflects audibility of speech presented at 45 dB HL. This same spectrum was applied to an input of 35 dB HL and to 50 dB HL. The amount of audibility as a percentage was determined for different bands of hearing loss in 5 dB increments for each of the two input levels. In addition, information was pro-

Student_____	Grade_School_____	Date_____

Loudness in dB HL	250	500	1000	2000	4000	8000 Hz
	Soft speech (35 dB HL)			Teacher voice (50 dB HL)		

Typical hearing children: Word recognition at 35 dB HL in quiet = 93-98%; in noise at 0 S/N = 8 6-94%.
Age 3-17 years   Word recognition at 50 dB HL in quiet = 9 3-100%; in noise at +5 S/N= 90-97% ; and 0 S/N = 89-9 6%.

0 **10** 95% audibility of speech energy perceived with hearing levels between 0 – 10 dB HL 64% at +10 S/N, 34% at 0 S/N[1,5]	0-20 dB HL should perceive 98% of speech sounds at a comfortable level in a quiet classroom and acceptable reverberation levels (35 dBA or less background noise in an unoccupied classroom & reverberation no greater than 0.9 sec[4])
75% audibility of speech energy perceived with hearing levels between 10 – 15 dB HL 44% at +10 S/N, 24% at 0 S/N	
15 60% audibility of speech energy perceived with hearing levels between 15 – 20 dB HL 29% at +10 S/N, 9% at 0 S/N	84% at +10 S/ N. 48% at 0 S/N
20 40% audibility of speech energy perceived with hearing levels between 20 – 25 dB HL 9% at +10 S/N, 0% at 0 S/N	95% audibility of speech energy perceived with hearing levels between 20 – 25 dB HL 81% at +10 S/N, 55% at 0 S/N
25 25% audibility of speech energy perceived with hearing levels between 25 – 30 dB HL 0% in any setting that is not quiet	81% audibility of speech energy perceived with hearing levels between 25-30 dB HL 67% at +10 S/N, 41% at 0 S/N
30 15% audibility of speech energy perceived with hearing levels between 30 – 35 dB HL 0% in any setting that is not quiet	60% audibility of speech energy perceived with hearing levels between 30-35 dB HL 46% at +10 S/N, 20% at 0 S/N
35 10% audibility of speech energy perceived with hearing levels between 35 – 40 dB HL 0% in any setting that is not quiet	45% audibility of speech energy perceived with hearing levels between 35 – 40 dB HL 31% at +10 S/N, 5% at 0 S/N
40	30% audibility of speech energy perceived with hearing levels between 40 - 45 dB HL 16% at +10 S/N, 0% at 0 S/N
45	

S/N means the loudness of the speaker's voice (i.e. teacher) over the background noise. 0 S/N = noise and voice are the same loudness.
FM negates the effects of background noise and distance and provides optimal access to verbal instruction in large and small groups.

Results of Functional Listening Evaluation (FLE): Type of speech materials used:

SPEECH PERCEPTION	Close: dB HL Quiet or +10 S/N	Close: dB HL Noise: -5 S/N +10 S/N	Distant: dB HL Quiet or +10 S/N	Distant: dB HL Noise: -5 S/N -10 S/N	Functional listening can be estimated in a sound suite via a 35 dB HL input to simulate listening a across room distance and 50 dB HL for listening at a closer distance (few feet).
Auditory + Visual					
Auditory Only					

Audibility represents the listening challenge caused by fragmented speech perception. Audibility should not be interpreted as speech perception, which shows well an individual recognizes the elements of speech that he perceives.

Recommended Hearing Technology/Accommodations:

AUDIBILITY Per the Audiogram above	Quiet No noise	+10 dB S/N Good classroom listening condition	0 dB S/N Very noisy classroom listening condition
Estimated Audibility Soft Speech			
Estimated Audibility Teacher's Speech			

Fig. 8.3 Speech Audibility Audiogram for Classroom Listening.

vided regarding the listening-in-noise ability of adults with speech inputs of 35 and 50 dB HL (Nelson, Anderson, Nie, & Katare, 2010). It can be assumed that children with hearing loss will not perform as well in terms of speech audibility as adults with normal hearing.

Audibility information does not take into account sloping hearing losses that are more than 10 dB greater in the high frequencies than in the low frequencies (Killion & Mueller, 2010). *Audibility should not be interpreted as speech intelligibility.* How persons use audible speech energy depends upon their knowledge of what is being talked about, the complexity of the information, and their ability to use context and communication repair clues to mentally fill in inaudible portions of speech so that spoken communication can be interpreted meaningfully. A person with 50 percent audibility may be able to identify 70 percent of single words and 95 percent of sentences (Miller, Heise, & Lichten, 1951). Audibility will be further compromised by the presence of varying background noise and classroom reverberation levels of 1.0 second or greater (Yang & Bradley, 2009), which can be negated by the use of FM during large group instruction. Understanding also may be enhanced by visual cues.

Picture Puzzle

To better understand the meaning of speech audibility, consider the analogy of trying to recognize the picture in a picture puzzle with only a limited number of pieces (**Fig. 8.4**):

1. How easy it is to recognize the subject of the puzzle depends on what pieces are missing and the complexity of the picture.
2. Perceiving speech is similar to a puzzle that is made up of text and missing pieces.
   - The solver has to understand the puzzle for well-known stories *and* for information with vocabulary that has never before been encountered—both with parts of the words missing throughout.
3. Unlike a picture puzzle, audibility and speech perception will be further compromised by the presence of varying background noise and classroom reverberation levels of 1.0 second or greater, although understanding will often be enhanced by visual cues.
4. Speech audibility is not the same as speech understanding. Speech audibility does, however, represent the student's listening challenge. The difference between audibility and un-

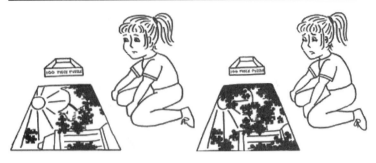

Fig. 8.4 Representation of 25 percent of puzzle pieces missing (left). Representation of 40 percent of puzzle pieces missing (right).

derstanding can be attributed to the student's level of language complexity, ability to attend (listen with focused effort) in challenging conditions, and skill at using context to build understanding.

5. The greater the gap between a student's audibility and speech understanding, the greater the support the student will require to prevent or minimize an increasing decline in academic performance over time.

6. To estimate a student's speech intelligibility for sentences and/or words under different listening conditions, a Functional Listening Evaluation (Johnson & VonAlmen, 1993) or a listening-in-noise assessment should be performed in a clinical setting at 0 S/N, +5 S/N, and +10 S/N at 35 dB HL and 50 dB HL.

◆ Functional Listening Evaluation (FLE) Under Varying Listening Conditions

The goal of the FLE is to determine, with a close estimate, how well the student is able to understand speech in a dynamic classroom setting. The FLE systematically obtains measures of how well a student can understand speech in quiet and in the presence of background noise, at close and far distances, and when watching the speaker's face and when not watching for visual cues. Preferably, a FLE is conducted in a student's classroom when the rest of the class is out of the room.

The FLE has long been a staple of educational audiology (Johnson & VonAlmen, 1993). Educational audiologists, speech-language pathologists, and teachers of the deaf and hard of hearing can perform a FLE. The professional most likely to perform a FLE typically depends on the staffing and workload assignment in each local school district. The FLE protocol indicates that listening should occur at distances of 3 feet and 12–15 feet (see **Fig. 8.5**). If it is possible to perform the FLE in the student's classroom, select the distance from the student's seat to where the teacher customarily stands as the near measure. A position across the room could be chosen to represent a peer responding to a question or the teacher wandering about the room, for the measure of listening at far distance. If it is not possible to perform the FLE in a classroom setting, use a therapy room or other available space. It is important to simulate typical classroom noise and distance conditions as closely as possible. Age-appropriate word lists or phrase lists are repeated under conditions of quiet and noise, watching and not watching the talker. The audiologist in a clinical setting can accomplish this same comparison task in a sound suite using 35 or 50 dB HL inputs and varying S/N levels. Results of the FLE are key to analyzing a student's access to verbal instruction under ideal and typical classroom conditions.

The Speech Audibility Audiogram for Classroom Listening (**Fig. 8.6**), completed for an example student, specifies the student's audibility and shows results of the FLE. Recommendations for hearing

	close/quiet or 50 dB HL	close/noise or 50 dB HL at +5 S/N	distant/quiet or 35 dB HL	distant/noise or 35 dB HL at +5 S/N
Auditory only				
Auditory and visual				

Fig. 8.5 FLE chart. S/N refers to the loudness of the speaker's (i.e., teacher's) voice over the background noise. Functional listening can be estimated in a sound suite via a 35 dB HL input to simulate listening across a room and a 50 dB HL input for listening at a closer distance (a few feet).

114 Handbook of Acoustic Accessibility

assistance technology (HAT) were developed using this information in **Fig. 8.6**. Thus, there is evidence beyond the student's hearing loss upon which to recommend the use of HAT to the school team. (Blank versions of the Speech Audibility Audiogram for Classroom Listening can be downloaded from http://successforkidswith hearingloss.com/resources-for-professionals#classroom-acoustics.)

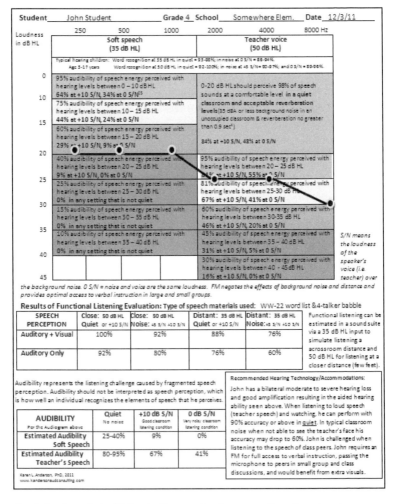

Fig. 8.6 Speech Audibility Audiogram for Classroom Listening, showing a specific student example. (Anderson & Arnoldi, 2011.)

◆ **Listening in Classroom Acoustic Conditions**

The classroom is a dynamic listening environment; therefore, the student's ability to perceive speech should be considered within the context of the acoustic conditions of the learning setting. The following brief explanations are provided to assist users of this handbook in explaining the potential effects of adverse acoustic conditions on student performance.

Reverberation

Background noise covers up talking so that it is mixed together, making it difficult to tell the words from the noise. Reverberation is different. Reverberation *smears* speech. This means that the last sound of the first word overlaps the first sound of the next word, making it hard to tell the words apart. The sentences in **Fig. 8.7** help to illustrate smearing. As reverberation time gets longer, the spaces between words get smaller and it takes more time and effort to figure out what was said. Not all reverberation smears speech. Some reverberation actually helps to reinforce speech, making the words easier to hear (see Chapter 3 of this handbook for more information). When you are outside, there are no walls for sound to bounce off, so you have to stand closer to people to hear them. You probably wish you had reverberation when you are outside.

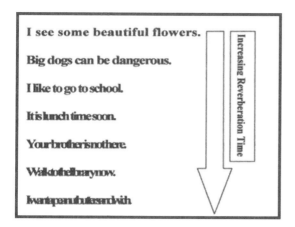

Fig. 8.7   Visual illustration of reverberation.

Background Noise

We refer to the difference between the loudness of the teacher's voice and the background noise as the *speech-to-noise* ratio, or S/N. If the teacher's voice is above the background noise, S/N is a positive (+) number, meaning a good hearing situation. If the teacher's voice is quieter than the background noise, S/N is a negative (−) number, meaning a poor hearing situation. An analogy of listening difficulty amidst noise is presented in **Fig. 8.8**. For best effect, look away from the chart and then quickly look back at it. At what level is it easy to read the sentence? Can you read all of the sentences? Think about how long and how much work it took to read the very bottom level.

Missing Bits and Pieces of Words

The simulation in **Fig. 8.9** shows how missing even a little content can make it more difficult to understand a message. Based on the Count-the-Dots Audiogram with an input of 45 dB HL, all of the sounds in words have been removed as though you had a 25 dB hearing loss (a mild hearing loss) and you were listening when it was just a little noisy. This is a common children's story. Can you guess what it is? If not, the answer follows in **Fig. 8.9**. Consider the effort you need to expend to puzzle out the words that are intended. The greater the effort expended to listen, the fewer the cognitive resources available to understand the message (Sarampalis,

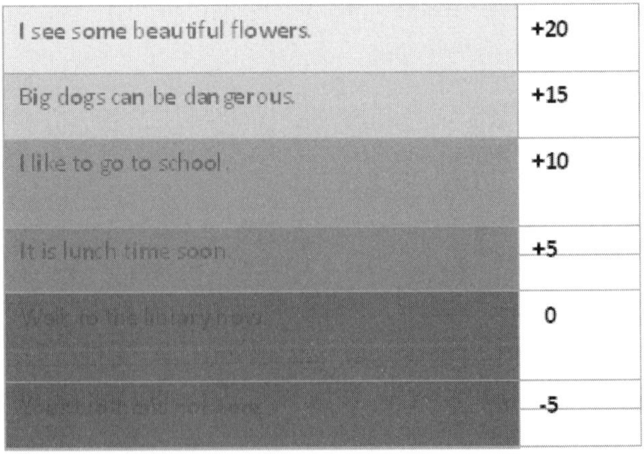

I see some beautiful flowers.	+20
Big dogs can be dangerous.	+15
I like to go to school.	+10
It is lunch time soon.	+5
Walk to the library now.	0
We get milk at the store.	-5

Fig. 8.8 An analogy of listening in noise.

> *Won upon a time a itty*
> *mow when to vit a untry*
> *mow. The untry mow*
> *live in a feel. EEE wuz lad*
> *toshee hi zittyfren.*
> *A too my ran abowda*
> *feel and lay untnoo.*

Fig. 8.9 Visual analogy of missing sounds in words due to a 20–25 dB hearing loss and typical classroom listening conditions: The Country Mouse and the City Mouse.

Kalluri, Edwards, & Hafter, 2009). Even appropriately fitted hearing aids do not "restore" normal hearing and listening ability.

◆ Verifying Effective Classroom Access: Input from Students and Teachers

So far, this chapter has presented information on how student audibility and speech perception can be estimated. These are both key aspects that affect how much and how well a student is able to listen in a typical classroom environment. The purpose of this section is to provide approaches to obtaining input from students and teachers that will identify how the student's ability to perceive speech is reflected under daily learning conditions.

Verifying Classroom Acoustics

Ultimately, it is the role of the audiologist working in the educational setting to measure the actual acoustics present in the learning environment. Refer to Chapter 4 in this handbook for specific information on how to perform classroom acoustic measurements.

Another approach, preferably used in combination with the above, is to ask the student to estimate the effects of classroom acoustics. One way is to ask the student to complete the *Estimating Classroom Noise Effects* form in **Fig. 8.10**. While not an actual measure, this form provides insights into the student's awareness of his or her acoustical learning setting and may act as a screen to identify the most important classrooms to measure for acoustic appropriateness. A second way is to administer the first page of the *Listening Inventory for Education—Revised (LIFE-R) Student Appraisal of Listening Difficulty* (http://successforkidswithhearingloss. com/tests/new-listening-inventory-for-education-revised-life-r). The Before-LIFE Questions for Students section asks the student to check off appropriate answers to the following questions:

1. Mark the items that best describe your classroom listening location.

Student_____Grade_____School_____		
The following questions are for students who are in a regular classroom setting.		
The questions do not apply to students in portable classrooms.		
Circle yes or no for each question.		
If you notice something at least every week or so, circle yes.		
If you notice something only once a month or so, circle no.		
1. Does your classroom have a hard floor surface (no carpeting on the floor)?	Yes	No
2. Do you notice when the fan noise starts for heating or air conditioning?	Yes	No
3. When your teacher is talking, are there times that you feel like you miss some of what he says because of noise made by other students in your class?	Yes	No
4. Do you notice when there is sound from the hallway outside of your classroom?	Yes	No
5. Do you notice the teacher's voice from the classroom next door to your classroom?	Yes	No
6. Would you say that your classroom is really large in size or has extra-high ceilings?	Yes	No
7. Are there whiteboards (or chalkboards) on more than one wall of your classroom?	Yes	No
8. When students with desks across the room from yours answer questions can you usually understand what they say without really working to listen and understand?	Yes	No
9. Does your teacher seem to need to talk pretty loud for everyone to hear in your classroom (not just a bit loud)?	Yes	No
10. Are there times you feel that you need to really work to listen so you don't miss part of what the teacher is saying?	Yes	No
Comments about how easy/hard it is for you to listen and understand in your classroom:		

If the total number of yes responses is 4 or more, this student may be experiencing listening difficulties in the classroom that are due in part to inappropriate classroom acoustics, warranting acoustical measurement.

Fig. 8.10   Estimating Classroom Noise Effects form.

2. What sounds (noises) do you hear when you are in the classroom?

3. When you are sitting in your usual location in the classroom, how well do you hear the teacher?

4. What is the best description of your teacher's location in the classroom when teaching (re: typical mobility)?

5. How well do you know when you did not hear or understand the teacher completely?

Verifying Student's Perception of Ability to Hear and Understand

The Functional Listening Evaluation (Johnson, Benson, & Seaton, 1997) is a measure used to estimate a student's ability to perceive speech. It is important to involve the student in the FLE by explaining why different distances, noise levels, and access to visual cues are used and how they will heighten his or her awareness of situations in which the most and least levels of challenge occur. Involving the student in the FLE as a learning opportunity is a first step toward raising the awareness needed for the student to recognize when it is important to self-advocate. Understanding the single-word or single-phrase stimuli used in the FLE is not the same as listening to connected speech at varying distances and noise levels and by different speakers. Only the student can provide information as to how well he or she is able to function under these conditions. To download the complete FLE, go to http://success forkidswithhearingloss.com/tests/tests-by-other-authors.

The LIFE-R Student Appraisal of Listening Difficulty (Anderson, Smaldino, & Spangler, 2011) (http://successforkidswithhearingloss. com/tests/new-listening-inventory-for-education-revised-life-r) presents 10 LIFE Classroom Listening Situations and 5 Additional/ Social Listening Situations in School. For each situation, the student must judge his or her level of difficulty in hearing and understanding. The sections are scored separately. The Student LIFE-R can be used as a pre-test and post-test after a trial with hearing assistance technology (HAT). In such a case the benefits of HAT are likely to be mainly in classroom listening situations. Although HAT may also improve performance in some of the additional listening situations, it is likely that self-advocacy skills and other access activities may need to be used to show benefit in these circumstances. After the additional listening situation questions, the Student LIFE-R provides a summary (**Fig. 8.11**) where the student and/or professional can identify all of the situations in which the student identified some level of listening challenge.

Verifying Teacher's Perception of a Student's Ability to Hear and Understand

Teachers are in a unique position to observe the student with hearing loss function in the classroom setting and to make judgments as to how the student's performance compares to students who do not have hearing loss. The *Listening Inventory for Education– Revised (LIFE-R) Teacher Appraisal of Listening Difficulty* (Anderson et al., 2011) can be used as a pre-test/post-test or as a stand-alone measure. It asks the teacher to rate a student's level of challenge when listening and learning for each of 15 questions. The responses are averaged and the resulting score identifies the level of challenge from "no listening challenges or very rare" to "almost always has listening challenges" (http://successforkidswithhearingloss .com/tests/new-listening-inventory-for-education-revised-life-r).

	_____'s most challenging listening situations
	1. Teacher talking in front of room
	2. Teacher talking with back turned
	3. Teacher talking while moving
	4. Student answering during discussion
	5. Hearing and understanding directions
	6. Other students making noise
	7. Noise outside of the classroom
	8. Multimedia (video, computer)
	9. Listening with fan noise on
	10. Simultaneous large and small group
	11. Cooperative small group learning
	12. Announcements
	13. Listening in a large room (assembly).
	14. Listening to others when outside
	15. Listening to students during informal social times
The more ☆'s the more difficult. No ☆ = no problem.	

Fig. 8.11 Of the 15 Listening Inventory for Education questions, these situations were rated as Always Difficult (☆☆☆), Mostly Difficult (☆☆), or Sometimes Difficult (☆).

◆ Monitoring Classroom Function over Time

Recent information (Yoshinaga-Itano, 2010) reviewed the developmental outcomes of children who are deaf or hard of hearing from age 12 months through 84 months with all levels of permanent hearing loss who use hearing aid or cochlear implant technologies. The results, depicted in **Fig. 8.12**, illustrate the changing student profile and the necessity of meeting the needs of today's students with hearing loss, who are more likely to attain typical academic performance than ever before. Almost half of all these students will have developmental language delays upon school entry and afterward. Almost 10 percent of those who enter school with age-appropriate skills develop a gap between their performance and grade-level expectations. Another 15 percent who enter school with developmental language delays will "catch up" and perform at grade-level expectations by about grade 2. Finally, about a third of the children will enter school with age-appropriate skills and will remain competitive with their class peers, at least into grade 2.

Thus, it is important to monitor the function of all students with hearing loss over time as classroom expectations and linguistic complexity change.

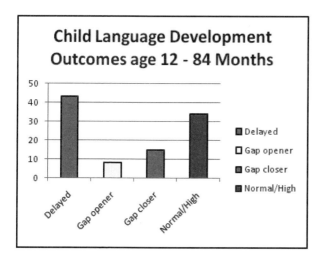

Fig. 8.12 Developmental outcomes of children who are deaf or hard of hearing (Yoshinaga-Itano, 2010).

Screening Instrument for Targeting Educational Risk (SIFTER)

SIFTER is composed of 15 questions on which the teacher compares the student's performance to that of class peers. There are 3 questions in each of the content areas of Academics, Attention, Communication, Class Participation, and School Behavior. The first SIFTER was developed in 1989 (Anderson, 1989) and is appropriate for use in grade 1 to the end of elementary school (grade 5 or 6). Due to SIFTER's successful widespread use, the Preschool SIFTER was developed in 1996 (Anderson & Matkin, 1996). It specifies Pre-Academics and Social Behavior areas more appropriate to young children and is designed to monitor children age 3 through kindergarten. Finally, the Secondary SIFTER was developed in 2004 (Anderson, 2004) for students in middle school/junior high through high school. The SIFTER and Secondary SIFTER screening checklists each result in a Pass, Marginal, or Fail score. The Preschool SIFTER identifies a child as at-risk or not at-risk for Social Behavior or Communication.

In a real-life example of tracking performance over time, a child with a mild bilateral sensorineural hearing loss (PTA 35 dB) was monitored at the end of kindergarten and again in first grade. In May of her kindergarten year, her teacher completed the Preschool SIFTER. The student passed the Pre-Academics, Attention, and Social Behavior sections and was found to be at risk for Communication and Class Participation. This same student entered grade 1, which is less visual and requires a higher level of listening accurately to follow directions, for early reading skill development, and for other capacities. In November of grade 1, the student's scores on the SIFTER were Pass for Attention and School Behavior, Marginal for Communication and Class Participation, and Fail in the area of Academics. This example underscores the need for and benefit of monitoring student function in the classroom, at least in the fall and spring of each year (mid-year is also recommended) so that prompt action can be considered if gaps in performance or other issues emerge.

Preschool SIFTER, SIFTER, and Secondary SIFTER can be downloaded from http://successforkidswithhearingloss.com/tests/tests-by-karen-anderson.

◆ The Important Role of Self-Advocacy Activities

Self-advocacy skills build on the development of communication skills and self-concept. Before individuals are willing to advocate for themselves, they need to have developed the perspective that they have a right and a responsibility to access the same information and to benefit from the same experiences as their peers. School programs that "take care" of students' accommodations and accessibility needs without directly involving and empowering them are counter-productive to the students' lifelong success. Students will not develop self-advocacy skills until they fully understand the importance of these crucial skills.

Verifying Self-Advocacy Skills (Obtaining Baseline and Measuring Growth)

To date, there has been little attention devoted to addressing students' self-advocacy skills and empowering them to recognize their right to equal access. Ultimately, these are skills with lifelong applications that should be learned and integrated into the student's lifestyle and interactions as early as possible. The following instruments have recently been developed to assist the student and school team in formulating student self-advocacy skill development.

Verifying the Student's Perception of Self-Advocacy

Upon revision of the Listening Inventory for Education, a component was added to assess students' perception of what they do when they have difficulty listening and understanding. The *LIFE-R Student Appraisal of Listening Difficulty: After-LIFE Questions for Students* instrument has six multiple-choice questions, each with five to eight possible answers (http://successforkidswithhearing loss.com/tests/new-listening-inventory-for-education-revised-life-r). The student is instructed to select all of the answers that apply. About half of the choices for each question indicate positive implementation of a self-advocacy strategy and about half indicate a lack of strategy or a negative response to the situation. These results, in addition to those for the other components of the LIFE-R Student Appraisal, provide a rich source of information for designing classroom accommodations, justifying the need for HAT, and developing student self-advocacy goals.

Verifying the Teacher's Perception of Self-Advocacy

The revision of the LIFE-R Teacher Appraisal (Anderson et al., 2011) also resulted in the inclusion of questions related to student self-advocacy. *LIFE-R Teacher Checklist: Self-Advocacy and Instructional Access* provides a space for the hearing professional involved in providing services to the student to specify the goals related to self-advocacy that have been included on the student's IEP. This is followed by eight questions specifying how often a student takes advantage of opportunities to self-advocate, including using strategic seating, a signal system, and positioning, as well as showing independence in caring for hearing technology. Requesting that teachers complete the Self-Advocacy and Instructional Access checklist is likely to raise the awareness of the teacher regarding self-advocacy and independence activities and expectations for students. (Download at http://successforkidswithhearingloss.com/tests/new-listening-inventory-for-education-revised-life-r.)

Development of Student Independence

IDEA Section 300.113 specifies that (a) each public agency must ensure that hearing aids worn in school by children with hearing impairments, including deafness, are functioning properly; and (b) each public agency must ensure that the external components of surgically implanted medical devices are functioning properly. At some point we must expect students to become fully independent in monitoring and taking care of their personal amplification devices. When does this start? What skills should be expected at what age? *Student Expectations for Advocacy & Monitoring Listening and Hearing Technology* or *SEAM for School Success* (see Appendix 8.1) (Anderson & Arnoldi, 2011) has been developed to provide a developmental hierarchy of expectations for student's independence with hearing technology and also some advocacy activities. It is recognized that some states may have specific requirements for monitoring frequency and reporting that do not align with these recommendations. Regardless, there is utility in having a developmental hierarchy of skills available to share with parents, students, and school professionals in those settings that lack substantial regular involvement of an educational audiologist.

◆ Audiologist's Role in Interpreting the Educational Effects of Hearing Loss

In many settings, the clinical audiologist in a community setting may be the most knowledgeable individual involved with the student regarding understanding the effects of hearing loss on education (see Chapter 9 of this handbook). In educational settings that employ audiologists, they are typically expected to be an important part of the team that will define the student's areas of educational need. In any setting, it is the role of the audiologist to advocate for the student's right to full access to verbal instruction and the need to monitor performance to ensure that full access is being achieved. Implicit in advocacy efforts is the knowledge of the student's acoustic learning environment and audibility/speech perception capabilities. This critical information enables the student to become fully independent with his or her amplification and hearing assistance technologies (HAT), a skill set that the audiologist is in a unique role to help build. Independence with HAT is a part of the overall right of the student to enjoy equal access and to advocate for his or her listening needs. Once again, access denied is opportunity denied. Success can be ensured only if performance is monitored and the results are considered periodically by all professionals involved with educating the student. The itinerant nature of the audiologist in the educational setting and the integral advocacy role of the audiologist in the clinical/community setting result in the audiologist's often being the logical choice to ensure that student performance is monitored over time. Finally, the audiologist is uniquely positioned to continually advocate for the student's right to full access to all educational opportunities within the educational setting—acoustically, socially, and educationally. Technology is one part of the solution to this need for full access. Sharing knowledge of the educational effects of hearing loss and advocating for a student's full access and ultimate lifelong independence is another.

◆ Appendix 8.1

Student Expectations for Advocacy & Monitoring Listening and Hearing Technology (SEAM)

The following expectations assume early identification of hearing loss, consistent amplification wear from infancy and supportive parent involvement in facilitating optimal listening and effective communication strategies. The age expectations are general indicators and should be adjusted as necessary due to lack of optimal audibility and/or early intervention services that include a focus on auditory independence.

Expected participation and/or skill to be consistently performed	Prior to school entry	1st day of school, PS/ Kdgn	By end of Kdgn	By end of gr 1	By end of gr 2	By end of gr 3	By end of gr 4	By end of gr 5	MS and HS
Wears hearing aid(s) or cochlear implant (CI) processor(s) full time.	X	X	X	X	X	X	X	X	X
Does self-test (baa baa, mmm mmm), listening to each device after it has been turned on.	X	X	X	X	X	X	X	X	X
Inserts (or attempts) earmolds and puts on hearing aid(s) or cochlear implant processor(s)	X	X	X	X	X	X	X	X	X
Recognizes that he needs to ask adult before device(s) are removed.	X	X	X	X	X	X	X	X	X
Knows that he is expected to report all issues with device(s).	X	X	X	X	X	X	X	X	X
Wears/brings hearing aid(s) or CI processor(s) to school every day.		X	X	X	X	X	X	X	X
Extra batteries brought to school and kept in a known location.		X	X	X	X	X	X	X	X
Participates in daily functional monitoring of device(s) with adult (battery check, visual inspection, listening check by normal hearing person, Ling* sound listening check).		X	X	X					
Student performs visual inspection of device(s) independently.			X	X	X	X	X	X	X
Student responsible for daily charging, proper use and careful handling of FM equipment.			X	X	X	X	X	X	X
Student requests use of the FM microphone by peers during group or social activities.			X	X	X	X	X	X	X
Student reminds teacher to use FM transmitter as appropriate.			X	X	X	X	X	X	X
Student understands how to appropriately let the teacher know when he is having trouble hearing or understanding.			X	X	X	X	X	X	
Student performs battery check independently.			X	X	X	X	X	X	X
Student cleans plugged earmold(s) (with supervision to grade 3).			X	X	X	X	X	X	X
Student is responsible to close classroom door if bothered by hallway noise.			X	X	X	X	X	X	X
Student knows that he must inform teacher when he is having difficulty understanding the teacher or other students speaking.			X	X	X	X	X	X	
Adult monitors devices 3 times per week, including Ling sound check.					X				
Two days per week the student does the Ling sound check with a classmate (3 & 10 feet).				X	X	X	X		
Student is allowed to remove device(s) in school for functional monitoring only.				X	X	X	X	X	X
Student responsible for recording results on the Daily Monitoring Worksheet.				X	X	X	X	X	X
Student actively uses communication repair strategies in the classroom and socially.				X	X	X	X	X	X
Student listens to self for Ling sounds daily.					X	X	X	X	X
Student will use a Dri-Aid kit if moisture accumulates in earmold tubing.						X	X	X	X
Student responsible for delivering the FM transmitter to teachers and advocating for use.						X	X	X	X
Adult monitors devices every 2 weeks, Ling sound check with classmate 2 days per week.						X			
Adult monitors devices every month, Ling sound check with classmate 2 days per week.							X		
Adult monitors devices every 3 months, including Ling sound check.									X
Student is responsible for promptly reporting technology problems, such as calling the audiologist directly.									X

*Ling sounds are presented at a typical conversational loudness with the student: aw, oo, ee, sh, s, m and acknowledging a silent trial visual cues. Child can repeat the sounds or point to a visual representation of the sounds. Personal/FM device(s) can be monitored at a distance of 3 and 10 feet in as quiet a setting as practical. The check at 3 feet can be eliminated as the student becomes more proficient at the Ling task.

IDEA Sec. 300.113. (a) Each public agency must ensure that hearing aids worn in school by children with hearing impairments, including deafness, are functioning properly. (b) (1) Each public agency must ensure that the external components of surgically implanted medical devices are functioning properly. *NOTE: It is recognized that some states may have specific requirements for monitoring frequency and reporting.*

Karen L. Anderson, PhD, 2011

References

Anderson, K. L. (1989). *Screening instrument for targeting educational risk.*

Anderson, K. L. (2004). *Secondary screening instrument for targeting educational risk.* Available at http://successforkidswithhearingloss.com/tests/tests-by-karen-anderson

Anderson, K. L., & Arnoldi, K. A. (2011). SEAM for school success. In *Building skills for success in fast-paced classrooms: Optimizing achievement for students with hearing loss* (p. 398). Butte, OR: Butte Publications.

Anderson, K. L. & Matkin, N. D. (1996). *Preschool screening instrument for targeting educational risk.*

Anderson, K. L., Smaldino, J. J., & Spangler, C. (2011). *Listening inventories for education—Revised.* Available at http://successforkidswithhearingloss.com/tests/new-listening-inventory-for-education-revised-life-r

Bodkin, K., Madell, J., & Rosenfeld, R. (1999). *Word recognition in quiet and noise for normally developing children.* AAA Convention, Miami, Poster Session.

Howard, A. (2010, March 9). National broadband plan takes shape with digital literacy corps. Available at http://www.huffingtonpost.com/alexander-howard/national-broadband-plan-t_b_492478.html

Johnson, C. D., Benson, P. V., & Seaton, J. (1997). Sentence and phrase lists (appendix section 15). In *Educational audiology handbook* (pp. 477–489). San Diego, CA: Singular.

Johnson, C. D., & VonAlmen, P. (1993). The functional listening evaluation. In *Educational audiology handbook* (pp. 336–339). (Revised in 2004 by C. D. Johnson.)

Killion, M., & Mueller, G. (2010). Twenty years later a new count-the-dots method. *Hearing Journal, 63*(1), 10, 12–14, 16–17.

Killion M., & Studebaker G. (1978). A-weighted equivalents of permissible ambient noise during audiometric testing. *Journal of the Acoustical Society of America, 63*(5), 1633–1635.

Miller, G. A., Heise, G. A., & Lichten, W. (1951, May). The intelligibility of speech as a function of the context of the test materials. *Journal of Experimental Psychology, 41*(5), 329–335.

Nelson, P., Anderson, E., Nie, Y., & Katare, B. (2010). Effect of reduced audibility on masking release for normal- and hard-of-hearing listeners. *Journal of the Acoustical Society of America, 127,* 1903.

Sarampalis, A., Kalluri, S., Edwards, B., & Hafter, E. (2009, October). Objective measures of listening effort: Effects of background noise and noise reduction. *Journal of Speech, Language, and Hearing Research, 52*(5), 1230–1240.

Yang, W., & Bradley, J. S. (2009, February). Effects of room acoustics on the intelligibility of speech in classrooms for young children. *Journal of the Acoustical Society of America, 125*(2), 922–933.

Yoshinaga-Itano, C. (2010). The longitudinal language learning of infants and children with hearing loss. ASHA Virtual EHDI Conference, October.

9   Acoustic Accessibility: The Role of the Clinical Audiologist

Jane R. Madell

◆ The Clinical Audiologist

The great majority of children with hearing loss will have a clinical/private audiologist who works at a hospital, clinic, or private office and with whom the family will have a comfortable and supportive relationship. Under ideal circumstances, the clinical audiologist will have identified the hearing loss, selected and monitored the hearing aids and/or cochlear implants to ensure acoustic accessibility throughout the frequency range, helped the family identify appropriate therapy and educational programs, recommended FM systems, and provided supportive counseling. As the child enters school, the clinical audiologist will work with the school staff to transfer some responsibilities to the educational audiologist at the school. Depending on the school system, this transfer may include all clinical audiology functions or just a portion, usually those directly related to assistive technology and classroom management. The educational and clinical audiologists will need to develop a good working relationship if the child is to function optimally. In communities where there is no educational audiologist, the clinical audiologist may have the additional responsibility of managing school technology and classroom accessibility. The purpose of this chapter is to discuss the critical role of clinical audiologists in securing and managing global acoustic accessibility for the children they serve.

◆ Selecting Appropriate Primary Technology

Hearing Aids

The importance of hearing well in all listening conditions and the advantage of FM systems in facilitating listening at a distance and in the presence of noise have been fully addressed in earlier chapters and need not be reviewed here. This discussion will focus on what is required for hearing technology to function optimally.

For FM systems to work appropriately, hearing aids must be carefully selected. The goal is a seamless connection between the FM and the hearing instruments. There are many factors involved in selecting the proper technology. First, the technology needs to compensate for the specific type of hearing loss. Aided thresholds must be tested to demonstrate hearing at sufficiently soft levels to confirm access to speech information throughout the frequency range, including high frequencies. Testing needs to be conducted in difficult listening conditions to determine what is and is not being heard. This includes assessing performance at normal and soft conversational levels in quiet and in noise (Dillon, Ching, & Golding, 2008; Madell, 2007, 2008a, 2008b; Stender, Appleby, & Hallenbeck, 2011). Testing will provide information about technology modifications that are needed to improve performance, including modifying the frequency response of hearing aids and cochlear implants, and modifying output to provide more gain in areas of the frequency spectrum where the child is not hearing specific phonemes (Hewitt, Madell, & Rotfleisch, 2011). Testing also will clearly indicate conditions where listening is a problem, and can justify the need for FM technology in a variety of educational and life situations.

In the selection of hearing aids for children, FM compatibility is critical. Even if an FM system is not going to be used on the day the hearing aids are dispensed, it should be assumed that a child will use FM during the life of the hearing aid. While classroom audio distribution systems (CADS) provide improved sound quality for children with typical hearing, children with hearing loss require personal FM systems to attain optimal listening (Anderson, Goldstein, Colodzin, & Iglehart, 2005). It is essential that hearing aids and cochlear implants be appropriately set to provide easy coupling to FM technologies, resulting in clear, undistorted signals.

Hearing aids for children should have direct audio input (DAI) capability and preferably use a size #13 or #675 battery so that they can be coupled to universal FM adaptors. Some FM manufacturers have systems that adapt to #312 batteries, but these are not universal and the school district may resist purchasing new equipment. Some hearing aids have a direct connect and come ready to plug into an FM adaptor. Others require that the hearing aid be returned to the manufacturer to be adapted. If a hearing aid is being recommended that does not directly connect to an FM system, the adaption apparatus should be ordered when the hearing aid is ordered so the hearing aid will be immediately available for FM use.

It is useful to consider FM audio shoe connectivity to the hearing aid. FM shoes that connect via the hearing aid battery door are easy to connect and easy to repair if needed. Changing the battery door can easily be accomplished in the audiologist's office. Other connectivity systems may require returning the hearing aid to the manufacturer if problems develop, resulting in time when the hearing aid is not available to the child.

Some manufacturers offer hearing aids with integrated FM. The advantage of these is that additional parts are not needed and the hearing aid is always FM ready. This can be a particular advantage for younger ears, as there will be fewer problems resulting from the FM boot's being attached and detached several times each day. The disadvantage is that if either the hearing aid or FM breaks, the entire system will need to be returned to the manufacturer for repair. In addition, some districts are very willing to purchase universal FM receivers that can be used by other students if needed (e.g., when students move out of the district) but may be uncomfortable purchasing an FM receiver that is hearing aid specific and can be used by only one student.

Some hearing aids are designed with automatic detection of the FM or DAI circuit. Others require changing programs. For the hearing aids that require switching programs, it is important to consider who will do the switching. Some children may easily be able to change technology programs, while others may not. We want to teach children to be independent and to take responsibility for their technology, so this issue may be something to consider. When programming the hearing aids, the audiologist may consider setting the FM program as the start-up program so that hearing aid programs will not have to be changed for FM use.

Selecting the Type of FM System for Use in All of the Child's Learning Environments: School, Home, and After-School Activities

There are several options to consider in selecting FM type. Anderson and others (2005) have demonstrated that CADS may not provide sufficient benefit for children with hearing loss. Personal FM systems are the system of choice for a child with hearing loss or auditory processing disorders.

Direct audio input (DAI) will plug into the hearing aid and should be seamless. The FM signal will be transmitted through the hearing aid so that the signal the child receives will have the same frequency response and gain as the hearing aid. The limit of what comes in through the FM will be affected by the bandwidth of the FM system. Hearing aids are being developed with expanded bandwidth in the high frequencies, providing important access to high-frequency phonemes. An FM with reduced bandwidth will not be able to make use of the expanded high frequencies of the new hearing aids. Current research (Madell, Lindley, & Bodkin, forthcoming) is evaluating how significant this bandwidth mismatch might be.

Neck loops may be selected if the hearing aid is not FM compatible. It is important to realize that the frequency response of the neck loop will limit the signal the child receives from the FM system, significantly reducing high-frequency gain. Another option for hearing aids that are not FM compatible is a desktop speaker system. Unlike DAI or neck loops, the desktop system does not seamlessly move with the child. If the child moves to another part of the classroom or to another room, she will need to carry the desktop speaker along. If a child turns his back on the desktop system to listen to something happening behind him, he will get a reduced signal. Some manufacturers use Bluetooth technology to pair devices, including FM receivers, to their hearing aids. These Bluetooth devices are manufacturer specific.

Cochlear Implants

Manufacturers of current cochlear implants set the implant to default at a 50/50 ratio, meaning that the sound coming from the FM microphone and that from the cochlear implant will be equally loud. This default is usually the appropriate setting. There may be some situations (such as a college lecture) where a 30/70 ratio (70 percent FM) might be more appropriate. The cochlear implant audiologist needs to check the settings to be sure that they meet requirements. If an induction coil is being used, either in school or outside of school, it is important to check the settings for the accessory ratio and the telecoil ratio on the cochlear implant. As with hearing aids, an induction loop will not provide as much high-frequency information as a direct connection will.

The type of FM system can make a significant difference. Recent research by Wolfe and colleagues (2009) compared several different FM systems and concluded that DAI resulted in better speech perception than MyLink connections, and that dynamic FM provided better performance than traditional FM. It is essential that the individual child be tested with the recommended FM system in several difficult conditions (soft speech and speech in noise) to be sure the system is working correctly and providing the expected benefit.

◆ Helping Families Accept the Need for FM at Home

Infants

Hearing aids do not provide sufficient benefit when the child and the primary talker are more than a few feet apart or when there is background noise. The more severe the hearing loss, the more that distance and noise are of concern. Families with children with newly identified hearing loss are likely to have a difficult time adjusting to the need for hearing aids and getting them to work appropriately. Managing the additional technology of an FM system may make things more difficult. This is often not a serious concern for an infant, who is typically very close to (in the arms of) the person speaking. However, once the infant starts to crawl, or is placed in an infant seat away from the primary talker, the signal will be degraded by distance and noise. Families need to understand the negative effect that distance and noise have on auditory brain development and language learning (Cole & Flexer, 2011). If parents can be made to understand the limits of hearing aids, they may be more willing to deal with the additional technology of an FM system. Infants, while in the car going to therapy, or even in a stroller with the parent several feet away, will receive significantly more auditory language input if the parent is using an FM system. Parents have reported that wearing the FM transmitter reminds them that they have to *talk, talk, talk*, and when they do not have it on, they feel less pressured to talk. This alone is a good reason to provide FM for every infant.

FM is especially important for infants with severe and profound hearing loss. Because of the difficulty of receiving a clear signal when they are even a few feet from the primary talker, FM should be considered at the initial fitting (Madell, 1992).

Toddlers

As toddlers develop, listening becomes more difficult. They are frequently not close to the person speaking, and they are often in situations with multiple talkers. Many toddlers start nursery school or are placed in a day care setting and will miss much if they do not have an FM system. It is usually not difficult to help parents understand the need for an FM system in a group setting. However, this understanding does not mean that the parents will be happy about it. Parents may feel that they should hide the hearing loss and may be concerned that the more equipment the child has, the more he will be considered "different" from his peers. It may be helpful to discuss the impact on the child of not hearing and not understanding what is being said in the group situation, and the negative effect this lack of auditory access has on language development and social skills.

After-School Activities

While the need for FM in school is clear, children also need to listen and hear outside of school. For children to succeed in sports, dance class, or religious training, they need to hear what is going on. Since these activities often take place at the end of the school day, we can expect that the child is already tired from listening all day long. Having to listen after school without the benefit of an FM system can add unnecessary pressure; the child will likely have to rely on visual cues and watch others to know what to do, which contributes to a feeling of incompetence. An FM system can significantly reduce the stress and effort of listening during after-school activities.

Using the FM at Home

Homes are noisy places. If there is one parent and one child at home, it may be possible to control the noise level, but once there are more than two people present, and especially if there are other children, it is not possible to control noise. The dinner table will be noisy, the backyard or playground will be noisy, and the living room will be noisy. An FM system can significantly improve listening in all these situations. Other children in the house can learn to use the transmitter, improving communication and providing more language input. The transmitter can be placed in front of the TV, facilitating understanding. Peers and friends are usually interested in learning to use the FM and, with some assistance, are usually cooperative about it.

Teaching Others to Use the FM

In any situation where the FM is being used, all users benefit from a lesson in FM procedures. First they need to understand why the FM is being used and the situations in which it should be used. They need to understand that the FM may not be needed in a quiet room where the child and the talker are sitting close together, but is needed when the child and talker are at a distance or when there is competing noise. The exception to this is a child with a profound hearing loss using hearing aids that do not provide input for soft speech. These children should be using FM as their primary means of amplification (Madell, 1992).Talkers often are advised that the FM should be on only when they are speaking to the child and should be turned off when they are addressing someone else. Specific settings for turning the FM on and off, or muting it, need to be made clear. On the other hand, there could be value in purposely letting the child "listen in" to the back-and-forth exchange between family members and, perhaps, between the teacher and another student. This overhearing is a valuable way to allow typical children to develop social competence and gain an understanding of the emotional exchanges between people. The challenge is to determine how to enable "listening in" to other conversations without compromising the child's independent work. The point is that we may be removing the child's opportunity to learn from other conversations by always turning off the FM mike when the child is not the direct target of the conversation.

◆ Monitoring FM Performance

Verification and Validation of FM Benefit

Refer to Chapter 7 in this handbook for a thorough discussion of the hearing assistance technology (HAT) guidelines (American Academy of Audiology, 2008). The guidelines identify fitting goals for hearing assistance technology to provide audibility and intelligibility in the following areas:

1. Speech recognition that is commensurate with performance in ideal listening situations
2. Full audibility of self and others
3. Reduced effects of distance, noise, and reverberation

It is essential to verify FM benefit. One should not assume that the FM is working simply because it is plugged in. The FM needs to be tested on the schedule recommended and checked every morning. The fact that the FM worked yesterday does not mean it is working today. Verification according to the manufacturer's protocol is always important to ensure that the child is receiving a consistent signal between the hearing aid and the FM system.

In addition to verification, validation is critical. Test booth validation should include performance with and without the FM system. Testing should include aided thresholds and thresholds with the FM system. If aided thresholds are not providing sufficient gain, the hearing aids will need to be adjusted prior to proceeding. While the FM system can improve performance, it cannot make up for a poorly fitted hearing aid. Speech perception testing should be performed using a test that is linguistically and age appropriate (Madell, 2008a). Testing should be conducted at normal (50 dB HL) and soft (35 dB HL) conversational levels in quiet and at a normal conversational level with competing noise, preferably four-talker speech babble (Madell, 2007, 2008a). See **Table 9.1** for an example of a test form that can be used to record test results.

Validation at Home and School

Validation should also be conducted in all situations in which the child is using the FM system, including at home and in school. At the very least, the FM system needs to be checked every day. It is not sufficient to ask the child if the technology is working. Many children with hearing loss are not able to accurately assess whether the system is working appropriately. The person with the microphone (parent, teacher, scoutmaster, etc.) should stand several feet away from the child to be sure the child is relying on the FM to receive the message and is not inadvertently receiving the signal only through the hearing aids. She may ask questions of the child to see if he is hearing. These should be questions that the child cannot anticipate and should be changed each day. Repeating the Ling sounds (*m*, *a*, *e*, *oo*, *sh*, *s*) in random order can also be a way to test FM performance.

Testing can also be conducted in the classroom to assess benefit. Johnson and Seaton (2012) have developed a Functional Listening Evaluation (FLE) (download from http://www.handsandvoices.org/pdf/func_eval.pdf) that assesses hearing up close and at a distance

Table 9.1   Test Form for Recording Speech Perception Testing Scores to Validate Technology Benefit

	Right Technology	Left Technology	Binaural	Binaural + FM
50 dB HL				
35 dB HL				
50 dB HL +5 SNR				

with and without the FM system. The FLE can be conducted in a classroom setting and provides important information about performance (**Table 9.2**). For information on using questionnaires to assess benefit, see Chapter 8 in this handbook.

◆ Helping Children Accept the Need for FM

When children are young, it does not usually occur to them to resist using technology. As children get older, acceptance can become more difficult. Children do not want to appear different from their peers and may resist calling attention to themselves. When children complain about needing to use technology, it is essential to give appropriate respect to their emotions. It is useful to confirm that it is not fair that the child has a hearing loss and has to use technology. This is a legitimate complaint. That being said, it is not an excuse to stop using the technology. If appropriate validation testing has been performed (**Table 9.1**), it is easy to show children the benefit of the FM. Most children are reasonable. Reviewing test results that show word recognition scores with and without FM with children is helpful in discussing FM's benefit. If older children are seriously resistant, it may be possible to negotiate FM classroom use only in connection with particular subjects where academics are a concern.

◆ Communicating with the School

Whether or not there is an educational audiologist in the school, the clinical audiologist will need to communicate with the school staff. Audiological reports need to be written in language that is meaningful to non-audiologists, and the report needs to be directed at school activities. The audiological diagnostics should evaluate and report on communication accessibility. The report needs

Table 9.2 A Functional Listening Evaluation Form

	Close Distance	**Far Distance**
Speech in quiet		
Speech in noise		

to carefully describe the child's acoustic accessibility/speech perception ability; if performance is described as good or excellent, the school will not be able to justify providing services. By testing speech perception in difficult listening conditions, a realistic picture of how a child will hear in school can be obtained, and thus services and accommodations can be justified.

As an example, **Table 9.3** presents speech perception test scores for a child with a moderately severe hearing loss. If testing had been conducted only at normal conversational levels in perfect quiet, results would be considered good for the right ear and binaurally, and fair for the left ear (**Table 9.4**) (Madell, Batheja, Klemp, & Hoffman, 2011). The need for services may not be clear. However, from test results for soft speech and for speech in noise, it becomes obvious that this child is struggling and will miss a great deal in the classroom. The need for auditory-based speech and language therapy is clear, as is the need for an FM system, a strategic seating plan, and the services of a teacher of the deaf and hard of hearing for previewing and reviewing academic material.

The clinical audiologist can make educational recommendations as they affect acoustic accessibility. This should certainly include specific recommendations about the need for an FM system with specific system suggestions, and may include recommendations about strategic seating, test accommodations, written assignments, and other pertinent concerns. Appendix 9.1 identifies some classroom accommodations that can be considered.

Table 9.3   Example of Speech Perception Test Scores for a Child with a Moderately Severe Hearing Loss (Madell, Batheja, Klemp, & Hoffman, 2011)

NU 6	Right Technology	Left Technology	Binaural	Binaural + FM
50 dB HL	84%	76%	84%	DNT
35 dB HL	64%	56%	60%	DNT
50 dB HL +5 SNR	DNT	DNT	56%	DNT

Table 9.4   Speech Perception Qualifiers

Excellent	90–100%
Good	80–89%
Fair	70–79%
Poor	<70%

◆ The Role of the Clinical Audiologist When There Is No Educational Audiologist

Unfortunately, at this time there are many school districts that do not have an educational audiologist on staff or as a consultant. As a result, there is no one in the school who is truly knowledgeable about acoustic accessibility and able to understand the needs of a child with hearing loss in the educational environment. School staff, like much of the public, may think that once a child has hearing aids or cochlear implants, all hearing-related problems are solved. The clinical audiologist can make a significant contribution to the child's management by stepping up as needed. It may not be possible for the clinical audiologist to attend IEP meetings in person, but he or she may be able to attend by phone, or at least provide written recommendations to parents and school in advance of the meeting. The audiological report should have a clear educational focus, with recommendations appropriate for school success. If there is no other advocate in the school, the clinical audiologist needs to help the school staff understand the effects of hearing loss on learning. This may include reporting on what reduced speech perception scores indicate, the stress of listening all day, the effect of reduced speech perception scores on testing, and suggestions for ensuring that the student with a hearing loss understands directions and assignments. It should not be assumed that a teacher knows how to use an FM system appropriately. Someone needs to carefully demonstrate the system's appropriate use, as well as troubleshooting and charging techniques. Teachers also need to know how to check that the FM is working each morning. An audiologist needs to be involved with this training.

The school staff cannot be expected to understand the negative effects of hearing loss on learning; it is the responsibility of audiologists to help the school staff understand the context of hearing loss in an educational setting. For young children, it may be behavior that is interfering with learning as children express their frustration. For older children, attentiveness may be questioned when, in fact, the child is having a problem hearing. Periodic in-services to staff are essential in order for school personnel to understand the challenges faced by students with hearing loss. Recordings of simulated hearing loss should be played and FM benefit should be demonstrated. By providing extensive information on individual children and the effect of their hearing loss on their education, we can help the school district personnel to understand the value of having an audiologist in the schools, perhaps leading to the hiring of an audiologist sometime in the future.

◆ Conclusions

The clinical audiologist has a significant role in managing a child with hearing loss. In the current climate, where many school districts do not have an educational audiologist on staff, the clinical audiologist has an expanded role. It is essential that the clinical audiologist take on more responsibility for managing school technology and assisting in classroom modifications. As we all know, it is not sufficient for a child to hear well in the test booth. For children to be successful, they need to hear well at home, at school, and in all after-school activities. Clinical audiologists are in a pivotal position to provide critical assistance to children with hearing loss to improve their prospects for school and life success.

◆ Appendix 9.1
Educational Recommendations

Personal FM Systems

1. FM for use during all academic subjects
2. Teacher training in appropriate use of the FM system—for both direct and incidental instruction
3. Troubleshooting information for FM system
4. Develop a system for the teacher to verify daily that the FM is working
5. Assign responsibility for daily charging of the FM system
6. Loaner FM available should the child's system break
7. Assign responsibility for returning the FM system to the factory for servicing over the summer

Classroom Noise Accommodations

1. No open classrooms
2. Select a classroom away from lunchroom, toilets, and playground to reduce noise
3. Carpeting in noisy places like the block corner
4. Acoustic tiles on walls and ceilings whenever possible
5. Tennis balls or hush-ups on chair and table legs to reduce noise
6. Monitor noise from heating and ventilation systems, and repair as needed

Strategic Seating

1. Seating in the front third of the classroom near the side to allow the student to see the teacher and also other students

2. Permission to move around the room as needed to hear and see

Teaching Accommodations

These accommodations can make a significant difference in a child's success.

1. Work to keep the classroom quiet to facilitate listening and learning for all children

2. Use "clear speech"; teacher's rate, pitch, and articulation can make speech easier to understand

3. Teacher faces student when speaking to facilitate receiving information

4. The classroom should encourage verbal communication with the opportunity for children to speak with each other

5. Repeat comments of other students into the FM microphone to be sure the student with hearing loss hears them

   • Use pass-around mike for FM to allow each student in the classroom to speak for herself

6. Call the student by name to be sure she knows you are talking to her

7. Confirm that the child with hearing loss hears and understands by asking questions (not "Did you hear that?" or "Do you understand?")

8. Reword, rather than repeat, if the message is not understood

9. Encourage the student to ask for clarification when information is not understood

10. Write assignments on the board or in a handout to be certain that the child receives the full assignment accurately

11. Consider assigning a buddy who can help the student with hearing loss get assignments, know what page to turn to, etc.

12. Observe what the student does and does not hear, and report this information to the audiologist, TOD, and speech-language therapist, to modify treatment
13. Activities requiring critical listening should be interspersed with activities that do not require intense listening
14. Provide listening breaks during the day to reduce the stress of listening

Test Accommodations

1. Testing should take place in a quiet room away from noise and interference
2. Directions should be provided clearly and the tester should verify that the student understands
3. Spelling tests should include a sentence so that words that sound similar will not be confused

Other Services to Be Considered

1. Students need regular audiological evaluations to monitor un-aided and aided hearing
2. Auditory-based speech-language therapy with a therapist experienced in working with children with hearing loss
3. Teacher of deaf or hard of hearing students to assess academic skills and preview and review academic material
4. Other tutoring as needed
5. Resource room as needed
6. All therapy or tutoring services should be conducted in a quiet place to facilitate learning
7. Develop a system for connecting the child's technology to computers or other media in "smart classrooms"
8. Team meetings for all staff working with the child with hearing loss to discuss concerns and plan remediation

References

American Academy of Audiology. (2008). *Clinical practice guidelines for remote microphone hearing assistance technologies for children and youth birth–21 years.* Available at http://www.audiology.org/resources/documentlibrary/Documents/HATGuideline.pdf

Anderson, K., Goldstein, H., Colodzin, L., & Iglehart, F. (2005). Benefit of S/N enhancing devices to speech perception of children listening in a typical classroom with hearing aids or a cochlear implant. *Journal of Educational Audiology, 12,* 16–30.

Cole, E., & Flexer, C. (2011). *Children with hearing loss: Developing listening and talking birth to six* (2nd Ed.). San Diego: Plural Publishing.

Dillon, H., Ching, T., & Golding, M. (2008). Hearing aids for infants and children. In J. R. Madell & C. Flexer, *Pediatric audiology: Diagnosis, technology and management.* New York, NY: Thieme Medical Publishers.

Hewitt, J., Madell, J. R., & Rotfleisch, S. (2011). Listen to the kids: Short course. AGBell Conference, July 21–23, Washington, DC.

Johnson, C. D., & Seaton, J. B. (2012). Functional listening evaluation. In *Educational audiology handbook* (2nd Ed., pp. 122–124). Clifton Park, NY: Delmar Cengage Learning.

Madell, J. R. (1992, April). FM systems as primary amplification for children with profound hearing loss. *Ear and Hearing, 13*(2), 102–107.

Madell, J. R. (2007, March-April). Using speech perception to maximize auditory function. *Volta Voices,* 16–20.

Madell, J. R. (2008a). Speech perception testing in infants and children. In J. R. Madell & C. Flexer, *Pediatric audiology: Diagnosis, technology and management.* New York, NY: Thieme Medical Publishers.

Madell, J. R. (2008b). Selecting appropriate technology: Hearing aids, FM, and cochlear implants. *Hearing Journal, 61*(11), 42–47.

Madell, J. R., Batheja, R., Klemp, E., & Hoffman, R. (2011, September). Evaluating speech perception performance. *Audiology Today.*

Madell, J. R., Lindley, G., & Bodkin, K. (Forthcoming). *FM bandwidth and its effect on speech perception.*

Stender, T., Appleby, R., & Hallenbeck, S. (2011). V&V and its impact on user satisfaction. *Hearing Review, 18*(4), 12–21.

Wolfe, J., Schafer, E. C., Heldner, B., Mülder, H., Ward, E., & Vincent, B. (2009, July–August). Evaluation of speech recognition in noise with cochlear implants and dynamic FM. *Journal of the American Academy of Audiology, 20*(7), 409–421.

Index

Note: Page numbers followed by *f* and *t* indicate figures and tables, respectively. Footnotes are indicated by *n.*